Examining and Solving Health Disparities in the United States:

Emerging Research and Opportunities

Cheryl Green
Southern Connecticut State University, USA

A volume in the Advances in Human Services and Public Health (AHSPH) Book Series

IGI Global
PUBLISHER of TIMELY KNOWLEDGE

Published in the United States of America by
IGI Global
Medical Information Science Reference (an imprint of IGI Global)
701 E. Chocolate Avenue
Hershey PA, USA 17033
Tel: 717-533-8845
Fax: 717-533-8661
E-mail: cust@igi-global.com
Web site: http://www.igi-global.com

Library of Congress Cataloging-in-Publication Data

Names: Green, Cheryl, 1968- author.
Title: Examining and solving health disparities in the United States : emerging research and opportunities / by Cheryl A. Green.
Description: Hershey, PA : Medical Information Science Reference, [2021] | Includes bibliographical references and index. | Summary: "This book provides awareness and discussion on the topic of inequities in healthcare that impact health disparities"-- Provided by publisher.
Identifiers: LCCN 2020043601 (print) | LCCN 2020043602 (ebook) | ISBN 9781799838746 (hardcover) | ISBN 9781799838753 (ebook)
Subjects: MESH: Health Status Disparities | Healthcare Disparities--economics | Health Services Accessibility--economics | Socioeconomic Factors | Minority Health | United States
Classification: LCC RA563.M56 (print) | LCC RA563.M56 (ebook) | NLM WA 300 AA1 | DDC 362.1089--dc23
LC record available at https://lccn.loc.gov/2020043601
LC ebook record available at https://lccn.loc.gov/2020043602

This book is published in the IGI Global book series Advances in Human Services and Public Health (AHSPH) (ISSN: 2475-6571; eISSN: 2475-658X)

British Cataloguing in Publication Data
A Cataloguing in Publication record for this book is available from the British Library.

Advances in Human Services and Public Health (AHSPH) Book Series

ISSN:2475-6571
EISSN:2475-658X

Editor-in-Chief: Jennifer Martin, RMIT University, Australia

MISSION

The well-being of the general public should be a primary concern for any modern civilization. Ongoing research in the field of human services and public healthcare is necessary to evaluate, manage, and respond to the health and social needs of the global population.

The **Advances in Human Services and Public Health (AHSPH)** book series aims to publish high-quality reference publications focused on the latest methodologies, tools, issues, and strategies for managing the health and social welfare of the public. The AHSPH book series will be especially relevant for healthcare professionals, policy makers, government officials, and students seeking the latest research in this field.

COVERAGE

- Social Work
- Domestic Violence
- Public Funding
- Youth Development
- Social Welfare Policy
- Medicare and Medicaid
- Health Policy
- Healthcare Reform
- Access to Healthcare Services
- Assistance Programs

IGI Global is currently accepting manuscripts for publication within this series. To submit a proposal for a volume in this series, please contact our Acquisition Editors at Acquisitions@igi-global.com or visit: http://www.igi-global.com/publish/.

The Advances in Human Services and Public Health (AHSPH) Book Series (ISSN 2475-6571) is published by IGI Global, 701 E. Chocolate Avenue, Hershey, PA 17033-1240, USA, www.igi-global.com. This series is composed of titles available for purchase individually; each title is edited to be contextually exclusive from any other title within the series. For pricing and ordering information please visit http://www.igi-global.com/book-series/advances-human-services-public-health/102256. Postmaster: Send all address changes to above address.

Titles in this Series

For a list of additional titles in this series, please visit:
http://www.igi-global.com/book-series/advances-human-services-public-health/102256

Examining Gun Regulations, Warning Behaviors, and Policies to Prevent Mass Shootings
Selina E.M. Kerr (Independent Researcher, UK)
Information Science Reference • ©2021 • 196pp • H/C (ISBN: 9781799839163) • US $195.00

Practical and Political Approaches to Recontextualizing Social Work
Jacques Boulet (Borderlands Cooperative, Australia) and Linette Hawkins (Action Research Issues Association, Melbourne, Australia)
Information Science Reference • ©2021 • 309pp • H/C (ISBN: 9781799867845) • US $195.00

Digital Services in Crisis, Disaster, and Emergency Situations
Lídia Oliveira (University of Aveiro, Portugal) Federico Tajariol (University Bourgogne Franche-Comté, France) and Liliana Baptista Gonçalves (University of Aveiro, Portugal)
Information Science Reference • ©2021 • 411pp • H/C (ISBN: 9781799867050) • US $195.00

Epidemiological Research Applications for Public Health Measurement and Intervention
Simon George Taukeni (University of Namibia, Namibia)
Medical Information Science Reference • ©2021 • 214pp • H/C (ISBN: 9781799844143) • US $295.00

Global Issues and Innovative Solutions in Healthcare, Culture, and the Environment
Mika Merviö (Kibi International University, Okayama, Japan)
Information Science Reference • ©2020 • 366pp • H/C (ISBN: 9781799835769) • US $195.00

Handbook of Research on Leadership and Advocacy for Children and Families in Rural Poverty
H. Carol Greene (East Carolina University, USA) Bryan S. Zugelder (James Madison University, USA) and Jane C. Manner (East Carolina University, USA)
Information Science Reference • ©2020 • 525pp • H/C (ISBN: 9781799827870) • US $265.00

For an entire list of titles in this series, please visit:
http://www.igi-global.com/book-series/advances-human-services-public-health/102256

IGI Global
PUBLISHER of TIMELY KNOWLEDGE

701 East Chocolate Avenue, Hershey, PA 17033, USA
Tel: 717-533-8845 x100 • Fax: 717-533-8661
E-Mail: cust@igi-global.com • www.igi-global.com

I thank God for being an ever-present comfort in my life. This book is dedicated to my loving husband, William Carl Green, and to our sons, Joshua William Green and Elijah Matthew Green. Thank you, each of you, for being a part of my life. Please know that your love is priceless to me.

Table of Contents

Foreword

When Dr. Green asked me to write this foreword, I was reminded of a time over 30 years ago when we were both undergraduate students at a small women's college in the northeast. Dr. Green was a nursing student, and she and her classmates had a heavy course load: classes, treatment plans, labs, and clinicals, all within one semester (I was a social work student and, while we were busy, no one seemed as stressed as the nursing students). We were good friends and lived next to each other in the dorm. Among many other things, we would talk about our classes—the professors we liked, the ones we weren't so sure about, the courses, different theories, and how all of this played out in the real world. One time, Dr. Green was talking about patient assessments. In one of her classes earlier that day, the professor talked about assessing a patient, looking at their skin, and referencing "pink" as being healthy. "What about brown-skinned people?" Dr. Green wanted to know. Certainly, Dr. Green pointed out, as nurses, not all the patients they would be treating would be White, and this assessment would not be relevant to People of Color. I don't think the professor had an answer for her. I also suspect that the professor never thought about the needs of Black, Latinx, Asian, or Indigenous patients because this lack of acknowledgement of people of color as patients is as old as our nation and continues to the present.

Most Americans are now familiar with the term "health disparities," however, many people are not familiar with how those disparities directly affect the lives of people of color: the statistics of more Black women dying in childbirth than White women, more Black and Latinx Americans dying from COVID-19 than White Americans. Most of us do not know the deep roots of these disparities or how to end them permanently.

This is why this book is so important. Healthcare practitioners and educators need to understand the history of health disparities, particularly the lack of accessibility based on systemic racism. Dr. Green explores this history and, equally important, solutions to end health disparities in the United States. As a healthcare practitioner and educator, Dr. Green understands that the medical field needs solutions as well as knowledge about its roots. It is telling that the title of Dr. Green's book includes the words "solving" and "opportunities." She has always been a great advocate of quality health care for all people, and this book is just one example.

Donna Morelli, JD, MSW

Preface

Health disparities have been a long-standing problem within the United States. Racial and ethnic minorities and the poor have, for years, encountered difficulty obtaining access to quality healthcare. The novel coronavirus, more commonly referred to as COVID-19, brought to the forefront these inequalities in access to healthcare by minority populations, such as Latinx and African Americans (Centers for Disease Control and Prevention, 2020), and lower-income Americans. As the death rate rapidly increased within these communities, health disparities in the United States could no longer be ignored. While access to health insurance can help, education that informs vulnerable populations on diet, exercise, the environmental impact of indoor and outdoor pollutants, genetics, and genomics can aid in lifestyle modification and stress reduction. However, without educating healthcare professionals about increasing their awareness of hidden biases, prejudgment, and discrimination, health disparities—despite innovative interventions and initiatives—will remain.

This book increases awareness and provides discussion on the topic of inequities in healthcare that impact health disparities. Pictures of people and neighborhoods are intentionally not used in this book. It is this author's intention to explore health disparities from a unifying perspective. Hence, images of nature that are representative of paths taken, and obstacles and journeys to be taken, will be symbolically used in the non-conventional exploration of this topic. It is only when open and honest dialogues are fostered in safe and neutral spaces that people can begin to understand why health disparities occur and how an increase in the awareness, education, and confrontation of discriminatory acts can help make changes at the organizational and, eventually, societal levels.

CHAPTER 1: DEFINING HEALTH DISPARITIES IN TERMS OF EQUITY

Disparities in health care have been a long-standing problem in the United States and internationally. Be it accessibility with regard to the ability to pay for services or the determination of who should receive care, fairness is not always a standard in providing quality health care. Hidden biases impact the type of care that people receive and, ultimately, affect mortality and morbidity rates among low-income and diverse populations.

CHAPTER 2: HISTORICAL OVERVIEW OF HEALTH DISPARITIES IN THE UNITED STATES

The evolution of health disparities in the United States carries with it a history of cultural bias, fear of the unknown, racism, sexism, and a desire to retain the status quo. However, as the United States population becomes increasingly more diverse, equitable treatment for all is imperative in health care.

CHAPTER 3: CULTURE, RACE, AND ETHNICITY

Culture, race, and ethnicity are uniquely different descriptions of people. The former reflects the traditions, faith, and belief systems in which humans are brought up, while the latter represent the physical characteristics and genetic variations they possess, as well as the geographic locations from which their families have descended. One's culture and racial/ethnic makeup positions them to view and experience the world and their immediate environment differently.

CHAPTER 4: PSYCHOLOGICAL IMPLICATIONS OF HEALTH DISPARITIES

As people of different religions, genders, races, ethnicities, cultures, and socioeconomic backgrounds seek entry into healthcare systems and receive poor-quality treatment that results from healthcare workers' conscious and unconscious biases, the psychological implications of these health disparities can be damaging. Linguistics—a cultural aspect of diversity—also impacts health care disparities because language barriers affect health literacy.

CHAPTER 5: ACCESSIBILITY FOR ALL

Health care is a human necessity to maintain mental and physical health in modern society. Accessibility to care is therefore the right of every human being.

CHAPTER 6: A SOLUTION

Solutions to end health disparities are complex and involve introspection and confronting one's perceptions of and beliefs about their fellow human beings who do not look like them. Universal design and cultural humility can help organizations examine how they welcome and treat people with different backgrounds.

CHAPTER 7: GRASSROOTS COMMUNITY COLLABORATIVES

A historical exploration of grassroots community initiatives involving health care in the United States is conducted. The potential effectiveness of past grassroots initiatives that could be implemented in the current healthcare environment is discussed.

CHAPTER 8: HOLDING HEALTHCARE SYSTEMS ACCOUNTABLE

Statistically, there are data that support the persistent existence of health disparities in the United States. Should healthcare systems and facilities be held accountable by their state and the federal government to show evidence of improvements in recognizing and resolving disparities experienced by vulnerable populations receiving care within their organizations? The answer to this question is yes.

REFERENCES

Centers for Disease Control and Prevention. (2020). *COVID-19 in racial and ethnic minority groups*. https://www.cdc.gov/coronavirus/2019-ncov/need-extra-precautions/racial-ethnic-minorities.html

Introduction

PURPOSE OF THE TEXTBOOK

The purpose of this textbook is to examine strategies for successful interventions in addressing health disparities and inequities in healthcare provided to affected populations. Populations deemed as being affected by health disparities within the United States include ethnic minority groups; older Americans; children; lesbian, gay, bisexual, and transgender people; and people in low-income households. The historical origins of health equity and disparities will be explored. This textbook is designed for students in healthcare professions such as public health, social work, and nursing. However, given the nature of the historical content, history and sociology departments would also benefit from introducing this textbook into their curriculums.

LEARNING OBJECTIVES

1. Identify the following populations of Americans that experience health disparities:
    a. Native Americans and Alaska Natives
    b. Hispanic/Latino Americans
    c. Native Hawaiians and Pacific Islanders
    d. Asian Americans
    e. African Americans
    f. Lesbian, gay, bisexual, and transgender people
    g. Older Americans
    h. Low-income households
2. Identify diseases that certain populations are more at risk for developing.
3. Consider how a lower socioeconomic status can impact health care access.

INTRODUCTION

Prejudgment

The act of *prejudgment* occurs when a person judges another before having evidence available that contradicts their assumptions or perceived beliefs about the other person. In healthcare, prejudgment can impact patient and provider relationships because presumptions are made by the healthcare providers about patients under their care in a relationship that can be perceived by the patients as authoritative. Kuiper (1983) suggests that it is important for health workers to be aware of their own prejudgments and how their prejudgment impacts healthcare and the healthcare system.

Implicit Biases

Implicit bias is an attitude or belief that is unconsciously associated with a specific group of people in varied life situations. Stereotyping is the driving force behind an implicit bias. Alspach (2018) identified patients who are at risk of experiencing implicit bias in healthcare as having any of the following attributes: non-English-speaking, obese, disabled, mentally ill, drug-addicted, non-White, female, non-heterosexual, or having acquired immune deficiency syndrome (AIDS) or low socioeconomic status.

Hall et al. (2015) reviewed 15 studies on implicit bias and found that there were four areas in which implicit bias impacted patients. These included patient health outcomes, patient–provider interactions, treatment adherence, and treatment decisions. FitzGerald and Hurst (2017) reviewed 3,767 articles and secured 42 articles that focused specifically on implicit biases in healthcare providers. Predominant themes within the 42 studies were biases regarding weight, race, ethnicity, gender, and age. All of the 42 studies reviewed by Hall et al. (2017) noted correlations between healthcare professionals' implicit biases and patients receiving quality, evidenced-based practice health care.

Dehon et al. (2017) conducted a systematic review on the objective disparities in the treatment and diagnoses received by ethnic minorities within emergency departments, and they examined implicit racial bias by physicians and the association of related clinical decisions made for patient care. They secured 1,154 articles, with nine meeting their criteria. Four criteria were applied in determining eligibility for inclusion of data: publication within peer-reviewed journals between 1998 and 2016; the inclusion of the Implicit Association Test as a measurement of implicit biases in the publications;

the inclusion of physicians; and assessment of physicians' clinical decision making. The findings were that in the treatment of such disease states and illnesses as pain, pediatric asthma, and acute myocardial infarction, the implicit preference for the delivery of health care to White people was preferred despite the physicians' specialty areas of practice. Evidence of poor quality of health care treatment decisions by physicians was noted in a study that found that White patients were more likely to receive thrombolysis for treatment of myocardial infarction. Current research indicates that while implicit biases do persist in healthcare environments with physicians' preference being given to the delivery of health care to White people, this bias does not impact clinical decision making.

Hidden Biases

Banaji and Greenwald (2013), in discussing hidden biases in their book entitled *Blindspot: Hidden Biases of Good People*, noted that after a lifetime of enculturation to attitudes about nationality, religion, age, gender, race, disability status, sexuality, ethnicity, and social class, everyone has hidden biases. *Hidden biases* are unconscious preferences that are held for a person or group of people. At a primitive level, the rationalization for hidden biases has been explained as people using biases against others as a means to protect themselves from a perceived threat. However, hidden biases impact how we interact with others, reject or accept them in the absence of knowing or understanding the person or people as individuals.

Self-talk is conducted daily on presumptions that we have of ourselves and others. With regard to hidden biases, if we consciously or unconsciously talk ourselves into believing that a group of people or a person is unworthy of the formation of a relationship with us, we can potentially translate this self-talk to insecurity and fear. Hence, racism and discrimination can emerge in our thought processes.

Institutional Racism in Organizations

Institutional racism, also referred to as *structural racism*, consists of hidden biases that are present within organizations. When institutional racism is not addressed in organizations, unhealthy work environments develop and are manifested by an inability to accept or maintain diversity within the workforce. As a result, employees with differing religions, gender, sexuality, age, ethnicity, race, and culture may leave the organization early after experiencing racism and discrimination because of the underlying organizational acceptance of hidden biases. Walter et al. (2017), in addressing hidden biases present in organizational systems, recommended the following:

1. Leadership has to recognize that they may be part of the problem
2. Leaders must openly share their intentions to address racism and institutional bias and the importance of cultural diversity
3. Create a senior management level position for a diversity officer
4. Implement strategies to implement training focused upon inclusivity, equity, and diversity
5. Develop succession plans of staff, membership, and leadership to ensure that the organization does not return to the status quo (Walter et al., 2017)

Diverse Workforces

In the United States, diversity in the workforce is increasing. A *diverse* workforce is one that is comprised of people of differing backgrounds and abilities (i.e., variations in physical and emotional abilities, religion, sexual orientation, ethnicity, gender, age, and socioeconomic status). There are now approximately 22 million Asians, 45.7 African Americans, 3.5 million Muslim Americans—with a projected growth of 8 million by 2050, 5.2 million Native Americans and Alaska Natives, and a projected 57 million Latinx (Hispanic/Latino people) in the workforce by 2035 (Industrial Safety and Hygiene News, 2020; Workplace Bullying Institute, 2020). However, despite the growth in diversity within the workplace, problems with racism and discrimination persist. Of the 60.4 million Americans that experience bullying in the workplace, Latinx people are bullied the most (Workplace Bullying Institute, 2020; Industrial Safety and Hygiene News, 2020).

Universal Design

Universal design is a concept that originated in architecture. Product designers, environmental researchers, architects, and engineers define universal design as the development of environments and products that can be used by all or at least most people whenever possible, without a necessity for specialized design or adaptation. In the making of designs that are accessible to all, from a societal perspective, the following seven principles of universal design must be applied: equitable use, flexibility in use, simple and intuitive use, perceptible information, tolerance for error, low physical effort, and size and space for appropriate use (University of North Carolina Charlotte, 2020).

Universal design has been incorporated into the United States Department of Labor's stance on the workplace. However, beyond workplace environments, universal design is representative of inclusivity. The following statement defines universal design from the perspective of the United States Department of Labor:

Universal Design (UD) is a strategy for making products, environments, operational systems, and services welcoming and usable to the most diverse range of people possible. Its key principles are simplicity, flexibility, and efficiency. And whether we realize it or not, most of us benefit from UD on a daily basis.

Originally developed in response to the needs of the aging population and people with disabilities, UD has much broader applicability. It increases ease of access to products, places, and services for multiple, diverse populations. Using UD means that facilities, programs, and services take into account the broad range of abilities, ages, reading levels, learning styles, languages, and cultures in their diverse workforce and customer base.

As a result, the Office of Disability Employment Policy has long promoted UD as an effective strategy for increasing the inclusion of people with disabilities, in both the workplace environment and the workforce system. (U. S. Department of Labor, 2020)

In application to health disparities and inequities, a universal design approach embraced by organizations that deliver healthcare to the poor and diverse populations could alleviate the burden of health disparities. Access to quality healthcare services provided by healthcare workers trained in universal design expectations of inclusivity makes organizations and the employees that work within them accountable. Universal design as a principle, at its core, is an ideal strategy in the restructuring of organizational systems that have both knowingly and unknowingly adapted hidden biases toward the populations of people that they serve.

Cultural Humility

The National Association of Social Workers defines *cultural humility* as the "attitude and practice of working with clients at the micro, mezzo, and macro levels with a presence of humility while learning, communicating, offering help, and making decisions in professional practice settings" (National Association of Social Workers, 2016, p. 16). The use of the term *cultural humility* came about as a response to the use of the term *cultural competence* by social service and healthcare workers (Nguyen et al., 2020). Cultural competence is an assumption of expertise about the culture of others. No one is an expert in all cultures, because cultures have sub-cultures whose norms will vary. Hence, cultural competence can easily lean toward the rationales of stereotypes.

Frameworks for cultural humility were initially proposed by the nursing and medical fields (Gottlieb, 2020). When applying cultural humility to working with diverse populations of people, it is an opportunity for one to explore their own perceptions of others and whether these perceptions are right or wrong. Ultimately, the determination of what is a stereotype or right and wrong information about culture can only occur when people approach one another as individuals without bias.

ALL PEOPLE MATTER: AN OVERVIEW OF HEALTH DISPARITIES

This section will provide an overview of diverse groups of people affected by health disparities within the United States. Groups of people to be discussed include Native Americans and Alaska Natives, African Americans, Asian Americans, Native Hawaiians, Pacific Islanders, Muslim Americans, Latinx (Hispanic/Latino) people, and lower-income non-Hispanic White households.

Native Americans and Alaska Natives

According to the Indian Health Service (IHS), the federal health program for American Indians (or Native Americans) and Alaska Natives, of the currently recognized 573 Alaska Native and American Indian tribes, health care services can be obtained through IHS healthcare facilities located in rural areas and reservations. There are an estimated 5.7 million Alaska Natives and American Indians in the United States according to the 2019 census; 2.56 million receive healthcare services provided by the federal government (IHS 2019; Office of Minority Health [OMH], 2021a). Mortality rates among American Indian and Alaska Natives are high in comparison to other Americans.

American Indians and Alaska Natives, on average, have a lower life expectancy of 5.5 years (73 years) in comparison to all races (78.5 years) in the United States. The leading causes of death (as of 2009–2011) are diabetes, malignant neoplasms, diseases of the heart, and unintentional injuries. American Indians and Alaska Natives surpass their fellow American citizens with high death rates due to intentional self-harm or suicide, unintentional injuries, assault or homicide, chronic liver disease, cirrhosis, chronic lower respiratory diseases, and diabetes mellitus (IHS, 2019). The 2020 census projection life expectancy for Alaskan Natives and American Indians is 78.4 years; 75.8 years for men and 81.1 for women (OMH, 2021a).

Since American Indians and Alaska Natives have a 5.5-times less-than-average life expectancy than any other Americans (as of 2009–2011), the IHS examined the age-adjusted mortality rates within their service areas, per 100,000 population. American Indians and Alaska Natives mortality disparity rates for all causes of death between the years 2009–2011 were 999.1 in comparison to all other races in America, at 747.0, a ratio of 1.3 (IHS, 2019). Measured specific causes of death of American Indians and all other races within the United States include (IHS, 2019): diseases of the heart 194.1 (other races 179.1, ratio 1.1); malignant neoplasm (cancer) 178.4 (other races 172.8, ratio 1.0); accidents (unintentional, including motor vehicle accidents) 93.7 (other races 38.0, ratio 2.5); diabetes mellitus (diabetes) 66.0 (other races 20.8, ratio 3.2); alcohol-induced deaths 50.0 (other races 7.6, ratio 6.6); chronic lower respiratory diseases 46.6 (other races 42.2, ratio 1.1); cerebrovascular diseases (stroke) 43.6 (other races 39.1, ratio 1.1); chronic liver disease and cirrhosis 42.9 (other races 9.4, ratio 4.6); influenza and pneumonia 26.6 (other races 15.1, ratio 1.8); drug-induced 23.4 (other races 15.3, ratio 1.5); nephritis and nephrotic syndrome (kidney disease) 22.4 (other races 15.3, ratio 1.5); intentional self-harm (suicide) 20.4 (other races 12.1, ratio 1.7); Alzheimer's disease 18.3 (other races 25.1, ratio 0.7); septicemia 17.3 (other races 17.3, ratio 10.6); assault (homicide) 11.4 (other races 5.4, ratio 2.0); and essential hypertension diseases 9.0 (other races 8.0, ratio 1.1).

Hispanic/Latino Americans

Hispanic/Latino Americans, defined as an ethnic group of American citizens, include people from Mexico, Central America, Spain, South America, Puerto

Rico, Cuba, Spain, and other Spanish origins and cultures. Race is not a factor, because Hispanic/Latino Americans have variations in skin, hair texture, and other characteristics. The current population of Hispanic/Latino people residing within the United States based on the 2019 US Census Bureau is 60.5 million: 61.4 Mexicans, 9.6% Puerto Ricans, 9.8% Central Americans, 6.4% South Americans, and 3.9% Cubans (OMH, 2021b).

In 2015, the average life expectancy for Hispanic/Latino people was noted to be 81.9 years of age; 79.6 for men and 84.1 for women. Comparatively, non-Hispanic White people have an average life expectancy of 79.8 years; 77.5 men and 82.0 for women. The current 2020 life expectancies estimates for Hispanic are 82.1 years of age; 79.9 years for men and 82.7 for women. Non-Hispanic Whites have an average life expectancy of 80.6 years of age; 78.4 for men and 82.7 for women (OMH, 2021b). The leading causes of illness and death in Hispanic/Latino people are diabetes, stroke, heart disease, unintentional injuries (accidents), and cancer. Other illnesses and diseases impacting Hispanic/Latino people include human immunodeficiency virus and autoimmune deficiency syndrome, asthma, liver disease, obesity, chronic obstructive pulmonary disease, and suicide. The low birth rate of infants most affects Puerto Rican mothers and their babies. Otherwise, rates of low infant births are lower in Hispanic/Latino populations when compared to non-Hispanic White populations (Office of Minority Health [OMH], 2019).

Fifty percent of Hispanic/Latino people are more likely than non-Hispanic White people to die from liver disease or diabetes (Centers for Disease Control and Prevention [CDC], 2015). Chronic liver disease was the fourth leading cause of death for Hispanic/Latino men that were aged 55–64 years in 2018 and the seventh cause of death within Hispanic/Latino populations (OMH, 2019). Hispanic/Latino people, in comparison to non-Hispanic White people, are 23% more obese, 28% less likely to have screening for colorectal cancer, and 24% more likely to have poorly controlled hypertension, 49% fewer have cancer, and 35% fewer have heart disease (CDC, 2015). It is important to note that there is a variation within data for preventative screenings and health risks among subgroups. For example, while Hispanic/Latino people smoke less than non-Hispanic White people (by 14%), 22% of Cuban males and 26% of Puerto Rican males smoke (CDC, 2015).

Native Hawaiians and Pacific Islanders

There are approximately 1.4 million Native Hawaiians and Pacific Islanders in the United States, with 355,000 Pacific Islanders and Native Hawaiians residing in Hawaii (OMH, 2021c). New York, California, Texas, Utah, Washington, Hawaii, Oregon, Florida, Utah, and Arizona have the highest populations of Native Hawaiians and Pacific Islanders. The three U. S. territories from the Office of Insular Affairs include Guam, the Northern Mariana Islands, and American Samoa. Their populations are 161,700 in Guam, 52,300 in Northern Marina Islands, and 57,000 in American Samoa. For other territories, the United Nations estimates the following populations of Native Hawaiians and Pacific Islanders: 18,000 in the Republic of Palau, 109,000 in the Federated States of Micronesia, and in the Marshall Islands. The life expectancy for Native Hawaiians and Pacific Islanders is 80.1 years; 77.7 years for men and 82.5 for women (CDC, 2020; United Nations Department of Economic and Social Affairs, 2020).

Native Hawaiians and Pacific Islanders have a high rate of tuberculosis (TB). In 2017, the incidence rate for TB was 19.1 in comparison to 0.5 for non-Hispanic White people. Obesity, alcohol consumption, and smoking were high as well. Native Hawaiians and Pacific Islanders have limited access to programs to help control and prevent cancer; hence cancer is one of their leading causes of death. Diabetes, cancer, stroke, heart disease, and unintentional injuries (accidents) are all leading causes of death for Native Hawaiians and Pacific Islanders. The percentage of diagnoses for asthma in 2015 was 13.9, compared to 13.5% for non-Hispanic White people, a ratio of 1.0. One year prior, in 2014, 30% of Native Hawaiians and Pacific Islanders, in comparison to non-Hispanic, were more likely to have asthma (CDC, 2017; OMH, 2017).

In Guam, from the years 2008–2012, the rate of cancers of all types, specifically for Micronesian populations, was 414.7. For Native Hawaiians in 2013–2015, it was 404.8, compared to 136.5 for non-Hispanic White people residing in Hawaii. Women residing in American Samoa are twice as likely to have a diagnosis of cervical cancer and also to die from this type of cancer, compared to non-Hispanic White people. Native Hawaiian men and American Samoan men are 2.4 times and 8 times more likely, respectively, to be diagnosed with liver cancer than their non-Hispanic White counterparts (OMH, 2020).

American Samoans were noted in 2014 to have the highest rates of diabetes than non-Hispanic White people, at 2.8, and among other Pacific Islander subgroups. The death rate for American Samoans related to diabetes is 6.2 higher than the national rate for non-Hispanic White people (OMH, 2019). The age-adjusted rate of diabetes diagnoses in 2018 for Native Hawaiians and Pacific Islanders for people of the age of 18-years and older was 19.8%.

Comparatively, for non-Hispanic White people, the age-adjusted percentage was 8.0%, with a combined ratio of 2.5 for both non-Hispanic White people and Native Hawaiians and Pacific Islanders (OMH, 2019).

There is presently limited data on heart disease available for Native Hawaiians and Pacific Islanders. Sub-populations tend to have variations in heart-related conditions. For example, people residing on the island of Guam in 2017 were noted to nearly be twice as likely to die from coronary heart disease in comparison to non-Hispanic White people nationally in the United States. However, in 2014, Native Hawaiians and Pacific Islanders were 10% more likely to be diagnosed with diabetes, in comparison to non-Hispanic White people (OMH, 2020).

Currently, there is no death rate data available regarding strokes among Native Hawaiians and Pacific Islanders. In 2014, Native Hawaiians and Pacific Islanders were nearly four times likely to have a stroke than non-Hispanic White people. For the sub-population of Northern Mariana Islanders, the death rate from stroke is 20% higher than the national rate for non-Hispanic White people (OMH, 2020). The age-adjusted stroke death rate per 100,000 in the year 2018 was 44.0 for Northern Mariana Islanders and 36.4 for U. S. national non-Hispanic White people, a ratio of 1.2 (CDC, 2019).

Asian Americans

There are approximately 18.9 million Asian Americans within the United States (OMH, 2021d; United States Census Briefs, 2012; United States Census Bureau, 2019). *Asian Americans* are Americans from the Indian subcontinent, Far East, and Southeast Asia. The following states had the highest populations of Asian Americans in 2019: Massachusetts, New York, Texas, New Jersey, California, Florida, Illinois, Hawaii, Washington, and Virginia (OMH, 2019). The average life expectancy for Asian Americans in 2020 was 80.7 years; 78.4 years for males and 82.7 years for females (OMH, 2021d)..

The leading causes of death for Asian Americans are stroke, cancer, and heart disease (National Vital Statistics Reports, 2019). For Asian American males over the age of 20 years, during the years 2013–2016, there was a 27.8% rate of hypertension, and for women, 24.2%. This data is based upon the intake of prescribed antihypertensive medications and measurements of increased blood pressure (CDC, 2018). In 2015–2017, 4.0% of Asian women over the age of 18 and 12.5% of males years smoked cigarettes; (CDC, 2018). Obesity for males over the age of 20 years in 2013–2106 was 11.7%, and for women over 20 years, 13.6% (CDC, 2018). In the year 2018, 8.3% of Asian Americans in varied age groups had poor or fair health (CDC, 2018).

Asian American and Pacific Islander women are two times more likely to be diagnosed with stomach cancer (per 100,000 women 2012–2016: 8.2 Asian and Pacific Islander women, 3.8 non-Hispanic White women) and 2.8 times more likely to die from stomach cancer. Asian and Pacific Islander women are less than 30% likely to be diagnosed with breast cancer than non-Hispanic White women (per 100,00 women in 2012–2016: 100.0 Asian and Pacific Islander women; 136.6 non-Hispanic White women). In 2012–2016, Asian and Pacific Islander men were twice as likely to be diagnosed with and die from stomach cancer (per 100,000 men in 2012–2016: 14.3 Asian and Pacific Islander men; 8.2 non-Hispanic White men) and 50% less likely to be diagnosed with prostate cancer (per 100,000 men in 2012–2016: Asian and Pacific Islander 55.6; 104.5 non-Hispanic White men). Asian and Pacific Islander women (per 100,000 women in 2012–2016: Asian and Pacific Islanders 7.4, non-Hispanic White women 3.7) and men (per 100,000 men in 2012–2016: Asian and Pacific Islanders 19.9, non-Hispanic white men 10.8) have nearly twice the incidence of inflammatory bowel disease (IBD) related cancers and liver cancers (National Cancer Institute, 2020; OMH, 2020).

Diagnosed cases of stroke for adults over the age of 18 years in 2018 for non-Hispanic Asian people is 2.7, non-Hispanic White people, 2.7, with a ratio of 1.0 (CDC, 2020). The age-adjusted stroke death rate per 100,000 during the year 2018 for Asian males was 32.1 (non-Hispanic White males 36.0, ratio 0.8) and non-Hispanic Asian women 28.7 (non-Hispanic white women 36.0, ratio 0.8). Asian Americans tend to be less likely to smoke cigarettes, not be overweight, and have lower rates of hypertension. Statistically, Asian Americans are 20% less likely to suffer a stroke that leads to death (CDC, 2019; OMH, 2020).

Asian Americans are 50% less likely than non-Hispanic White people to die from heart disease. The age-adjusted coronary heart disease percentage for Asian Americans over the age of 18 years in 2018 was 4.4%, 5.8% for non-Hispanic White people, a ratio of 0.7 (CDC, 2020). Per 100,000, the age-adjusted rates for heart disease in 2017 were 108.1 for non-Hispanic Asian and Pacific Islander men and 67.7 for women. For non-Hispanic White women, the age-adjusted rate for heart disease in 2017 was 131.9, 214.0 for men. The ratio of non-Hispanic Asian and Pacific Islanders to non-Hispanic White people_was 0.5 (CDC, 2019).

African Americans

There are approximately 40.6 million African Americans in the United States. In 2019, the ten states with the largest populations of African Americans were Maryland, Florida, Louisiana, New York, Texas, California, Virginia, Illinois, Georgia, and North Carolina. The average life expectancy for African Americans is 77 years, 74.0 for men and 79.8 for women. Comparatively, for non-Hispanic White people, the average life expectancy is 80.6 years, 78.4 for men and 82.7 for women (OMH, 2021e).

African Americans have a higher death rate in comparison to non-Hispanic White people for diabetes, influenza, cancer, heart disease, pneumonia, stroke, the human immunodeficiency virus, and acquired immunodeficiency syndrome. Additionally, rates of obesity and hypertension tend to be higher (age-adjusted percentage for African Americans over age 20 years in 2013–2016 with a BMI of 25 or greater: 80.6 for women and 70.6 for men). The age-adjusted percentage for African Americans 20 years of age and older with hypertension, in the years 2013–2016, was 42.9% for women and 41.8% for men. Non-Hispanic White men 20 years of age and older have an age-adjusted rate for hypertension of 31.1; women, 27.0. Elevated cholesterol levels and high blood pressure that are associated with obesity increase the risks of African Americans for diabetes, stroke, and heart disease (CDC, 2019; Agency for Healthcare Research and Quality, 2020).

Cigarette smoking is a lifestyle choice that can significantly impact risks for cancer, heart disease, and respiratory illnesses. The age-adjusted percentages for African Americans over the age of 18 years who actively smoked cigarettes in 2018 were 11.6% for women (non-Hispanic White women, 14.4) and 17.6% for men (non-Hispanic White men, 16.7). The percentage of non-Hispanic White people that have received advice to stop smoking for their health over the age of 18 years in 2016 was 67.9%; 60.7% for African Americans. The age-adjusted percentages for African Americans over the age of 20 years with an elevated cholesterol level in 2013–2016 were 23.8% for women and 24.3% for men; 31.6% for non-Hispanic White women, and men, 33.6%. The percentage of African Americans that received cholesterol screening in the last five years as of 2017 was determined to be 90%.1; 87.3% for non-Hispanic White people (Agency for Healthcare Research and Quality, 2020; CDC, 2020).

The age-adjusted percentages for African Americans diagnosed with coronary artery disease for ages 18 years and older is 5.4% (non-Hispanic White people, 5.8%). The death rate per 100,000 in 2017 for African Americans was 264.8, and for non-Hispanic White people, 214.0, a ratio of 1.2 (CDC, 2019, 2020). With regard to asthma, approximately 2.6 million African Americans reported having been diagnosed with asthma in 2015. African American children, in comparison to non-Hispanic white children, are four times more likely to be hospitalized for treatment of asthma. In 2014, African Americans were nearly three times more likely to die of asthma-associated complications. Children in homes that fell below the poverty level were found to have high levels of the nicotine byproduct cotinine. Secondhand smoke exposure from tobacco also placed African American children at an increased risk for developing acute lower respiratory tract infections (OMH, 2018).

Sixty percent of African Americans are likely to be diagnosed with diabetes, and, in 2017, twice as likely to die from complications associated with diabetes. African Americans with diabetes in 2016 were 2.3 times more likely to undergo surgery for lower limb amputations and 3.5 times likely to receive a diagnosis of end-stage renal disease in comparison to non-Hispanic White people (CDC, 2018, 2019; OMH, 2019). Women of African American descent are twice as likely to have a stroke in comparison to non-Hispanic White women, and African Americans are 60% more likely to die from a stroke than non-Hispanic White men. Overall, African Americans are 50% more likely to develop cerebrovascular disease (stroke; OMH, 2020).

Of any ethnic or group, African Americans are the most likely to die from cancer. This includes most major cancers and all cancers combined. For example, in 2012–2016, African American women were 40% more likely than non-Hispanic White women to die from breast cancer and 2.2 times to die from stomach cancer. In comparison to non-Hispanic White men, African American men have a lower five-year cancer survival rate and are 1.2–1.7 times more likely to be newly diagnosed with prostate or colon cancer, 2.5 times more likely to die from stomach cancer, and twice as likely to die from prostate cancer (CDC, 2020; National Cancer Institute, 2020; OMH, 2020).

The infant mortality rate for African Americans is 2.3 times that of non-Hispanic White people. African American infants in 2017 were 3.8 times more likely to die from complications associated with low birth rates and twice as likely to die from sudden infant death syndrome. Pregnant African American women in 2017 were 2.3 times more likely to have no prenatal care or to obtain prenatal care late in their pregnancies (CDC, 2019; OMH, 2019).

Lesbian, Gay, Bisexual, and Transgender

The *lesbian* (i.e., primary attraction of female to female), *gay* (i.e., primary attraction to people of the same gender), *bisexual* (i.e., attraction to both male and female), and *transgender* (i.e., people who no longer identify with their sex assigned at birth; LGBT) population was traditionally incorporated into the statistics of health disparities for the diverse races, ethnicities, social classes and religions with which they identified with. Gender and sexual orientation data were not commonly collected in all states in national surveys taken in the United States. Current research suggests that, because of societally based discrimination with which the LGBT population must contend, LGBT people have a high rate of suicide (Haas et al., 2011; Mullaney, 2016), mental health issues (Cortes et al., 2019; Drescher et al., 2018; King & Richardson, 2017), and substance abuse (Kerr & Oglesby, 2017; Williams & Fish, 2020).

The CDC, in describing health disparities among LGBT youths, uses the terms *lesbian*, *gay*, *bisexual*, *transgender*, and *queer* or *questioning* (LGBTQ). People identifying as queer identify as a member of the LGBT community. The term *queer* can be used in reference to the LGBT community itself, while the term *questioning* is the individual's exploration of gender expression, sexual orientation, and gender identity (CDC, 2019). According to a 2017 Youth Risk Behavior Survey completed by the CDC, health disparities were noted to exist with approximately 2.6 million sexual minority students. These health disparities included suicide (48% LGB, compared to 13% heterosexual), illicit drug use (23% LGB, compared to 12% heterosexual), being bullied at school (33% LGB, compared to 16% heterosexual), feeling hopeless or sad (63% LGB, compared to 28% heterosexual), misuse of prescription opioids (24% LGB, compared to 13% heterosexual), and being forced to have sex (22% LGB, compared to 5% heterosexual).

Transgender youths are more likely than their heterosexual (*cisgender*) peers to engage in high-risk sexual behaviors and, as a result, require testing for sexually transmitted infections and the human immunodeficiency virus. Transgender youths are more likely to engage in substance use and experience violence victimization. The latter information on transgender youth comes from a questionnaire distributed to high school students identifying as transgender in 19 school districts in ten states: Wisconsin, Rhode Island, Maine, Vermont, Michigan, Massachusetts, Delaware, Hawaii, Colorado, and Maryland. Data gathered from select school districts within these ten states indicate that 1.8% of high school students identified as transgender (Johns et al., 2018).

Older Americans

The Older Americans Act (OAA) was passed by the United States Congress in 1965 as a means to address the limited community-based social services available to older Americans. Research and grants supported the training of personnel to work with older populations, health promotion, and developmental planning within communities. The OAA was reauthorized most recently in March of 2020 by Congress. This reauthorization will remain current through 2024. Nationally, a network of approximately 56 state agencies, 20,000 providers, 618 agencies on aging, one Native Hawaiian organization that represents 400 tribes, and 281 tribal organizations offer services to older Americans as a part of the OAA (Administration for Community Living, 2020).

In regard to evidence-based health promotion disease prevention programs, in the 2006 amendments to the OAA, all 50 United States can design programs that improve the quality of life and health for older Americans under Title III (English language proficiency) and Title IV (access to educational programs). Programs that address substance abuse, diet and nutrition, fall prevention, depression, chronic disease self-care practices, and increasing physical activity can all be designed and implemented by the individual states, nationally. The goal of the National Council on Aging is to improve the quality of life for 40 million older Americans by the year 2030 (Administration for Community Living, 2020; National Council on Aging, 2020).

Low-Income Households

In 2019, the median American income per household was $68,703. Comparatively, in 2018, the median income was $64,324; a total increase of $4,379 (6.8%). This was the fifth decline in poverty in the United States since the publication of trending of poverty data began in 1959 (United States Census Bureau, 2020). Asian, Black, Hispanic, and White households all had increased income in 2019. In 2018–2019, Americans experienced increased income as follows: Asians decreased from 2.8% to 7.3%, Blacks 2.0% to 18.8%, Hispanics 1.8% to 15.7%, and Whites 1.0% to 9.1% (United States Census Bureau, 2020).

Figure 1. Quality, evidenced-based health care benefits all people

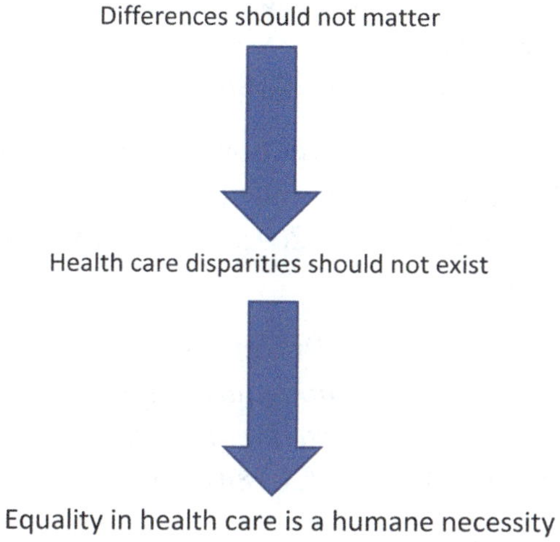

REFERENCES

Administration for Community Living. (2020). *Older Americans Act*. https://acl.gov/about-acl/authorizing-statutes/older-americans-act

Agency for Healthcare Research and Quality. (2020). *National healthcare quality and disparities report: Data query—Table 7_5_1_4_2.1*. Retrieved January 8, 2021, from http://nhqrnet.ahrq.gov/inhqrdr/data/query

Alspach, J. G. (2018). Implicit bias in patient care: An endemic blight on quality care. *Critical Care Nurse*, *38*(4), 12–16. https://doi.org/10.4037/ccn2018698

Banaji, M. R., & Greenwald, A. G. (2013). *Blindspot: Hidden biases of good people*. Delacorte Press.

Centers for Disease Control and Prevention. (2015). *Hispanic health: A la buena salud!* Retricvcd January 25, 2021, from https://www.cdc.gov/vitalsigns/hispanic-health/

Centers for Disease Control and Prevention. (2017). *Summary health statistics: National health interview survey*. Retrieved January 1, 2021, from https://minorityhealth.hhs.gov/omh/browse.aspx?lvl=4&lvlid=75

Centers for Disease Control and Prevention. (2018a). *National diabetes statistics report, 2017*. https://www.cdc.gov/nchs/data/nvsr/nvsr68/nvsr68_09-508.pdf

Centers for Disease Control and Prevention. (2018b). *Table 19: Current cigarette smoking among aged 18 and over, by selected characteristics—United States, average annual, selected years 1990–1992 through 2015–2017.* https://www.cdc.gov/nchs/data/hus/2018/019.pdf

Centers for Disease Control and Prevention. (2018c). *Table 22: Hypertension among adults aged 20 and over, by selected characteristics—United States selected years 1984–1994 through 2013–2016.* https://www.cdc.gov/nchs/data/hus/2018/022.pdf

Centers for Disease Control and Prevention. (2018d). *Table 26: Normal weight, overweight, and obesity among adults aged 20 and over, by selected characteristics—United States, selected years 1988–1994 through 2013–2016.* https://www.cdc.gov/nchs/data/hus/2018/026.pdf

Centers for Disease Control and Prevention. (2018e). *Table P-1a: Age-adjusted percent distribution (with standard errors) of respondent-assessed health status, by selected characteristics—United States, 2018.* https://ftp.cdc.gov/pub/Health_Statistics/NCHS/NHIS/SHS/2018_SHS_Table_P-1.pdf

Centers for Disease Control and Prevention. (2019a). *Adolescent and school health: Health disparities among LGBTQ youth.* Retrieved January 1, 2021, from https://www.cdc.gov/healthyyouth/disparities/health-disparities-among-lgbtq-youth.htm

Centers for Disease Control and Prevention. (2019b). *Births final data for 2017 national vital statistics reports.* https://www.cdc.gov/nchs/data/nvsr/nvsr67/nvsr67_08-508.pdf

Centers for Disease Control and Prevention. (2019c). *Health United States, 2018.* https://www.cdc.gov/nchs/data/hus/hus18.pdf

Centers for Disease Control and Prevention. (2019d). *Infant mortality statistics from the 2017 period linked birth/infant death data set.* https://www.cdc.gov/nchs/data/nvsr/nvsr68/nvsr68_10-508.pdf

Centers for Disease Control and Prevention. (2019e). Article. *National Vital Statistics Reports, 68*(9). https://www.cdc.gov/nchs/data/nvsr/nvsr68/nvsr68_09-508.pdf

Centers for Disease Control and Prevention. (2019f). Table 1: Deaths—Leading causes for 2017. *National Vital Statistics Reports, 68*(6), 1–76. https://www.cdc.gov/nchs/data/nvsr/nvsr68/nvsr68_06-508.pdf

Centers for Disease Control and Prevention. (2020a, November). *Health of Asian or Pacific Islander population*. Retrieved January 15, 2021, from https://www.cdc.gov/nchs/fastats/asian-health.htm

Centers for Disease Control and Prevention. (2020b). *Summary health statistics: National health interview survey*. Retrieved from https://www.cdc.gov/nchs/nhis/shs/tables.htm

Cortes, J., Fletcher, T. L., Latini, D. M., & Kauth, M. R. (2019). Mental health differences between older and younger lesbian, gay, bisexual, and transgender veterans: Evidence of resilience. *Clinical Gerontologist*, *42*(2), 162–171. https://doi.org/10.1080/07317115.2018.1523264

Dehon, E., Weiss, N., Jones, J., Faulconer, W., Hinton, E., Sterling, S., & Choo, E. K. (2017). A Systematic review of the impact of physician implicit racial bias on clinical decision making. *Academic Emergency Medicine*, *24*(8), 895–904. https://doi.org/10.1111/acem.13214

Drescher, C. F., Lopez, E. J., Griffin, J. A., Toomey, T. M., Eldridge, E. D., & Stepleman, L. M. (2018). Mental health correlates of cigarette use in LGBT individuals in the Southeastern United States. *Substance Use & Misuse*, *53*(6), 891–900. https://doi.org/10.1080/10826084.2017.1418087

FitzGerald, C., & Hurst, S. (2017). Implicit bias in healthcare professionals: A systematic review. *BMC Medical Ethics*, *18*, 19. https://doi.org/10.1186/s12910-017-0179-8

Gottlieb, M. (2020). The case for a cultural humility framework in social work practice. *Journal of Ethnic and Cultural Diversity in Social Work*. doi:10.1080/15313204.2020.1753615

Haas, A. P., Eliason, M., Mays, V. M., Mathy, R. M., Cochran, S. D., D'Augelli, A. R., Silverman, M. M., Fisher, P. W., Highes, T., Rosario, M., Russell, S. T., Malley, F., Reed, J., Litts, D. A., Haller, E., Sell, R. L., Remafedi, G., Bradford, J., Beautrais, A. L., Brown, G. K., … Clayton, P. J. (2011). Suicide and suicide risk in lesbian, gay, bisexual, and transgender populations: Review and recommendations. *Journal of Homosexuality, 58*(1), 10–51. doi:10.1080%2F00918369.2011.534038

Hall, W. J., Chapman, M. V., Lee, K. M., Merino, Y. M., Thomas, T. W., Payne, K., Eng, E., Day, S. H., & Coyne-Beasley, T. (2015). Implicit racial/ethnic bias among health care professionals and its influence on health care outcomes: A systematic review. *American Journal of Public Health*, *105*(12), e60–e76. https://doi.org/10.2105/AJPH.2015.302903

Indian Health Service. (2019). *Disparities*. Retrieved February 1, 2021, from https://www.ihs.gov/newsroom/factsheets/disparities/

Johns, M. M., Lowry, R., Rasberry, C. N., Dunville, R., Robin, L., Pampati, S., Stone, D. M., & Mercer Kollar, L. M. (2018). Violence, victimization, substance use, and suicide risk among sexual minority high school students: United States, 2015–2017. *Morbidity and Mortality Weekly Report*, *67*(43), 1211–1215. https://doi.org/10.15585/mmwr.mm6743a4

Kerr, D. L., & Oglesby, W. H. (2017). LGBT populations and substance abuse research: An overview. In J. VanGeest, T. Johnson, & S. Alemagno (Eds.), *Research methods in substance abuse*. doi:10.1007/978-3-319-55980-3_16

King, S. D., & Richardson, V. E. (2017). Mental health for older LGBT adults. *Annual Review of Gerontology & Geriatrics*, *37*(1), 59–75. https://doi.org/10.1891/0198-8794.37.59

Kuiper, J. P. (1983). Prejudgment and healthcare: Ethics of the helping relationship. *Psychiatric Annals*, *13*(6), 473–482. https://doi.org/10.3928/0048-5713-19830601-07

Mullaney, C. (2016). Reshaping time: Recommendations for suicide prevention in LGBT populations—Reflections on "Suicide and suicide risk in lesbian, gay, and transgender populations: Review and recommendations" from *Journal Homosexuality 58*(1). *Journal of Homosexuality*, *63*(3), 461–465. https://doi.org/10.1080/00918369.2016.1124712

National Association of Social Workers. (2016). *Standards and indicators for cultural competence in social work practice*. Author.

National Cancer Institute. (2020). *SEER cancer statistics review (CSR) 1975–2016*. Retrieved January 10, 2021, from https://seer.cancer.gov/archive/csr/1975_2016/index.html#contents

National Council on Aging. (2020). *Older Americans Act*. Retrieved February 8, 2021, from https://www.ncoa.org/public-policy-action/older-americans-act/

Nguyen, P. V., Naleppa, M., & Lopez, Y. (2020). Cultural competence and cultural humility: A complete practice. *Journal of Ethnic and Cultural Diversity in Social Work*. doi:10.1080/15313204.2020.1753617

Office of Minority Health. (2017a). *Asthma and Native Hawaiians and Pacific Islanders*. United States Department of Health & Human Services. Retrieved January 2, 2021, from https://minorityhealth.hhs.gov/omh/browse.aspx?lvl=4&lvlid=75

Office of Minority Health. (2017b). *Asthma and African Americans*. United States Department of Health & Human Services. Retrieved January 28, 2021, from https://minorityhealth.hhs.gov/omh/browse.aspx?lvl=4&lvlid=15

Office of Minority Health. (2019a). *Diabetes and African Americans*. United States Department of Health & Human Services. Retrieved February 17, 2021, from https://minorityhealth.hhs.gov/omh/browse.aspx?lvl=4&lvlid=18

Office of Minority Health. (2019b). *Diabetes and Native Hawaiian/Pacific Islanders*. United States Department of Health & Human Services. Retrieved January 25, 2021, from https://minorityhealth.hhs.gov/omh/browse.aspx?lvl=4&lvlid=78

Office of Minority Health. (2019c). *Profile: Hispanic/Latino Americans*. United States Department of Health & Human Services. Retrieved February 10, 2021, from https://minorityhealth.hhs.gov/omh/browse.aspx?lvl=3&lvlid=64

Office of Minority Health. (2020a). *Cancer and African Americans*. United States Department of Health & Human Services. Retrieved February 11, 2021, from https://minorityhealth.hhs.gov/omh/browse.aspx?lvl=4&lvlid=16

Office of Minority Health. (2020b). *Cancer and Native Hawaiian/Pacific Islanders*. United States Department of Health & Human Services. Retrieved February 18, 2021, from https://minorityhealth.hhs.gov/omh/browse.aspx?lvl=4&lvlid=76

Office of Minority Health. (2020c). *Heart disease and Native Hawaiian/Pacific Islanders*. United States Department of Health & Human Services. Retrieved February 16, 2021, from https://minorityhealth.hhs.gov/omh/browse.aspx?lvl=4&lvlid=79

Office of Minority Health. (2020d). *Stroke and Native Hawaiian/Pacific Islanders*. United States Department of Health & Human Services. Retrieved February 9, 2021, from https://minorityhealth.hhs.gov/omh/browse.aspx?lvl=4&lvlid=88

Office of Minority Health. (2020e). *Stroke and African Americans*. United States Department of Health & Human Services. Retrieved February 17, 2021, from https://minorityhealth.hhs.gov/omh/browse.aspx?lvl=4&lvlid=28

Office of Minority Health. (2021a). *Profile: American Indian/Alaska Native. United States Department of Health & Human Services*. Retrieved May 2, 2021, from https://minorityhealth.hhs.gov/omh/browse.aspx?lvl=3&lvlid=62

Office of Minority Health. (2021b). *Profile: Hispanic/Latino Americans. United States Department of Health & Human Services*. Retrieved May 1, 2021, from https://minorityhealth.hhs.gov/omh/browse.aspx?lvl=3&lvlid=64

Office of Minority Health. (2021c). *Profile: Native Hawaiians/Pacific Islanders. United States Department of Health & Human Services*. Retrieved May 2, 2021, from https://minorityhealth.hhs.gov/omh/browse.aspx?lvl=3&lvlid=65

Office of Minority Health. (2021d). *Profile: Asian Americans. United States Department of Health & Human Services*. Retrieved May 2, 2021, from https://minorityhealth.hhs.gov/omh/browse.aspx?lvl=3&lvlid=63

Office of Minority Health. (2021e). *Profile: African Americans. United States Department of Health & Human Services*. Retrieved May 2, 2021, from https://minorityhealth.hhs.gov/omh/browse.aspx?lvl=3&lvlid=61

United Nations Department of Economic and Social Affairs. (2020, December). *Population facts: Policies on spatial distribution and urbanization have broad impacts on sustainable development*. https://www.un.org/development/desa/pd/sites/www.un.org.development.desa.pd/files/undes_pd_2020_popfacts_urbanization_policies.pdf

United States Census Briefs. (2012, March). *The Asian population: 2010*. https://www.census.gov/prod/cen2010/briefs/c2010br-11.pdf

United States Census Bureau. (2017). *Selected population profile in the United States*. Retrieved February 27, 2021, from https://data.census.gov/cedsci/table?q=ACSSPP1Y2017.S0201&t=006%20-%20American%20Indian%20and%20Alaska%20Native%20alone%20%28300,%20A01-Z99%29%3A009%20-%20American%20Indian%20and%20Alaska%20Native%20alone%20or%20in%20combination%20with%20one%20or%20more%20other%20races%20%28300,%20A01-Z99%29%20%26%20%28100-299%29%20or%20%28300,%20A01-Z99%29%20or-%20%28400-999%29%3A012%20-%20Asian%20alone%20%28400-499%29%3A050%20-%20Native%20Hawaiian%20and%20Other%20Pacific%20Islander%20alone%20%28500-599%29%3A060%20-%20Native%20Hawaiian%20and%20Other%20Pacific%20Islander%20alone%20or%20in%20combination%20with%20one%20or%20more%20other%20races%20%20%28500-599%29%20%26%20%28100-299%29%20or%20%28300,%20A01-Z99%29%20or%20%28400-999%29%3A400%20-%20Hispanic%20or%20Latino%20%28of%20any%20race%29%20%28200-299%29%3A451%20-%20White%20alone,%20not%20Hispanic%20or%20Latino%3A453%20-%20Black%20or%20African%20American%20alone,%20not%20Hispanic%20or%20Latino&tid=ACSSPP1Y2017.S0201

United States Census Bureau. (2019). *Asian American and Pacific Islander Heritage Month 2019*. Retrieved January 23, 2021, from https://www.census.gov/newsroom/facts-for-features/2019/asian-american-pacific-islander.html

United States Census Bureau. (2020). *Income and poverty in the United States: 2019*. Retrieved January 17, 2021, from https://www.census.gov/library/publications/2020/demo/p60-270.html

United States Department of Labor. (2020). *Office of Disability Employment policy: Universal design*. Retrieved January 29, 2021, from https://www.dol.gov/agencies/odep/program-areas/employment-supports/universal-design/resources

University of North Carolina Charlotte. (2020). *Universal design*. Retrieved February 22, 2021, from https://teaching.uncc.edu/services-programs/teaching-guides/online-and-blended-courses/universal-design

Walter, A. W., Ruiz, Y., Tourse, R. W. C., Kress, H., Morningstar, B., MacArthur, B., & Daniels, A. (2017). Leadership matters: How hidden biases perpetuate institutional racism in organizations. *Human Services Organizations: Management, Leadership, & Governance, 41*(3), 213–221. doi:10.1080/23303131.2016.1249584

Williams, N. D., & Fish, J. N. (2020). The availability of LGBT-specific mental health and substance abuse treatment in the United States. *Health Services Research, 55*(6), 932–943. https://doi.org/10.1111/1475-6773.13559

ADDITIONAL READING

HealthyPeople.gov. (2020). *Lesbian, gay, bisexual, and transgender health*. Retrieved January 15, 2021, from https://www.healthypeople.gov/2020/topics-objectives/topic/lesbian-gay-bisexual-and-transgender-health

Chapter 1
Defining Health Disparities in Terms of Equity

ABSTRACT

Disparities in healthcare limit accessibility to care among affected populations and can include imbalances in the equitable achievement of optimal health. These imbalances occur as a result of differences that others have in financial means, education, culture, age, race, gender, sex, ethnicity, and religion. Consequentially, as health disparities persist among populations, mortality and morbidity rates reflect these inequities in health care. Hence, human life is quantified by geographic location, skin color, language, poverty, and an inability to culturally assimilate with majority populations. Hidden biases overshadow the pricelessness of human life, disease management, and disease prevention. Chapter 1 provides an overview of what encompasses health disparities and how equity is involved. Vulnerable populations within the United States are examined, and hidden biases are discussed as factors that impact the achievement of equitable healthcare.

LEARNING OBJECTIVES

1. Explore the meaning of the phrase "health disparity" in terms of the provision of quality, evidenced-based care to all United States residents.
2. Consider how inequality in the distribution of health care can have a negative impact on persons of low socioeconomic status, the insured, underinsured, and those with no insurance.

DOI: 10.4018/978-1-7998-3874-6.ch001

3. Explain the vision and mission of the Healthy People Initiative and what populations have been identified as potential vulnerable recipients of suboptimal health care.

Reflective Quote: "If I would have known of the inequalities in healthcare earlier, I could have educated and advocated for others without fear of recourse."

INTRODUCTION

Health equity was defined by the Healthy People Initiative 2030 (Office of Disease Prevention and Health Promotion [ODPHP], 2019; ODPHP, 2021) as the ability of all people to attain the highest level of health. Disparities in health care arise when there is an imbalance between opportunities to achieve optimal health care in terms of access, education, and financial means. However, the difficult subject of health disparities and their historical origins demonstrate that culture, race, and ethnicity may contribute significantly to health crises among minority groups in the United States (US). However, Americans who are poor, underinsured or uninsured, or live in either rural areas or low-income urban areas also experience health disparities related to their **socioeconomic status (SES)**. The resolution of health care disparities is possible when the psychology of disparity is examined and health care problems are explored in relation to the **biopsychosocial** (a model that combines social, psychosocial, and biological factors in understanding human beings) differences of human beings.

The socioeconomic complexities of health disparities impact access to care. For patients in the US who do not have insurance or maintain full-time employment, paying for health care can place households in financial turmoil. The degenderizing of health care has also been a factor in health disparities because health care research was traditionally male-oriented.

EVERY PERSON'S HEALTH IS IMPORTANT

The Healthy People Initiative began in 1979 under the leadership of physician Julius Benjamin Richmond. Dr. Richmond was a public health administrator and pediatrician, as well as a Harvard professor of health policy. In service to Americans' education about health and well-being, Dr. Richmond was the first national director of the Head Start Program, and developed health reports on smoking and health in 1979, which eventually led to the Healthy People report (ODPHP, 2019; Harvard T.H. Chan School of Public Health, 2021).

Since its inception in 1979, the Healthy People Initiative set forth by the US government's Department of Health and Human Services (DHHS) under the ODPHP has, for every ten years, researched and collected data that identify health disparities. Vulnerable populations affected by these health disparities and by acute and chronic areas of disease progression, can potentially shorten lifespans. Hence, Healthy People has become a valuable initiative that has the potential to increase the quality and length of life for all Americans.

The **vision,** or plan for the future, of Healthy People 2030 is to have "a society in which all people can achieve their full potential and well-being across the lifespan." The **mission,** or assignment to be carried out, is "to promote, strengthen, and evaluate the nation's efforts to improve the health and well-being of all people" (ODPHP, 2021). Overarching goals set forth by Healthy People 2030 include such issues as the prevention of premature death, injury, disability, and disease; the attainment of health equity and health literacy; and the elimination of health disparities. The five overarching goals of Healthy People 2030 are:

1. Attain healthy, thriving lives and well-being free of preventable disease, injury, and premature death.
2. Eliminate health disparities, achieve health equity, and attain health literacy to improve the health and well-being of all.
3. Create social, physical, and economic environments that promote attaining the full potential for health and well-being for all.
4. Promote health development, healthy behaviors, and well-being across all life stages.
5. Engage leadership, key constituents, and the public across multiple sectors to take action and design policies that improve the health and well-being of all. (ODPHP, 2021)

Healthy People 2030 has identified seven foundational principles to guide decision-making about helping Americans achieve optimal health. These seven principles include:

1. The health and well-being of all people and communities is essential to a thriving, equitable society.
2. Promoting health and well-being and preventing disease are linked efforts that encompass physical, mental, and social health dimensions.

3. Investing to achieve the full potential for health and well-being for all provides valuable benefits to society.
4. Achieving health and well-being requires eliminating health disparities, achieving health equity, and attaining health literacy.
5. Healthy physical, social, and economic environments strengthen the potential to achieve health and well-being.
6. Promoting and achieving health and well-being nationwide is a shared responsibility that is distributed across the national, state, tribal, and community levels, including the public, private, and not-for-profit sectors.
7. Working to attain the full potential for health and well-being of the population is a component of decision-making and policy formulation across all sectors. (ODPHP, 2021)

Given that, with the Healthy People Initiative, we have had a societal framework for the identification of and potential end to health disparities since 1979, it would logically seem that lifespans of Americans should have increased during this time, and disparities involving chronic disease states, injuries, mental health, suicide, cancer, cardiac disease, and premature deaths for younger and older Americans should have improved. While we have seen a gradual increase in the lifespans of all Americans, disparities remain based on SES, racial-ethnic background, and the geographic location in which people reside (urban, suburban, or rural areas). These disparities can also be improved. However, that would require all Americans to recognize why they exist and how to resolve them together.

An Evolving Nation: 2014 to 2060

The US population is projected to increase from 319 million to 417 million between the years 2014 and 2060. By 2060, approximately one in five US residents will be foreign born, and by 2044, it is estimated that half of all Americans will belong to an ethnic-minority group. By 2030, one in five will be older than 65 years of age (Colby & Ortman, 2015). With an aging population, more retirements will occur and there will likely be more older adults in the US than children. It is also projected that there will be more deaths than births (Vespa et al., 2020).

Approximately 175 million Americans reside within small metropolitan and suburban areas, with 98 million located in urban centers and 46 million in rural areas (Parker et al., 2018). Since the year 2000, the population in urban areas has increased by 1.6 million people. This population growth in cities has been attributed to the movement of new migrants to the regions and to the fact that there are more births in urban areas. In the suburbs, population increase has been caused by domestic and international migration. During the same period, rural areas saw a *decline* in their population, by 380,000, with 950,000 people expected to leave rural communities, and 600,000 new migrants (Parker et al., 2018).

THE SOCIOECONOMICS OF HEALTH CARE

The affordability of health care complicates equity with regard to access to health services. The US currently operates under what is called a multi-payer system. Within **multi-payer systems**, health care is jointly paid for by customers and the employers for which they work; money is collected by insurance companies for the reimbursement of services provided to customers by care providers. Multi-payer systems' payers include the government (i.e., the Medicare or Medicaid programs) and private insurance companies.

Single-payer systems, in contrast to multi-payer systems, have one organization that obtains financial fees from consumers and pays for health care services. The single-payer system is purported by supporters, such as the non-profit advocacy group Physicians for a National Health Program (PNHP, 2019), to decrease administrative costs and ease the burden of multiple insurances being billed by healthcare facilities and providers. Arguably, one must consider the financial sustainability of a single-payer system, especially one sustained by government funding from taxpayers in the US.

US Health Expenditures

In the US, the per capita expenditure for health care in 2018 was $11, 172, while total national health spending reached $3.6 trillion dollars, or 17.7% of gross domestic product (GDP; Centers for Disease Control and Prevention [CDC], 2019). Nationally, expenditures for hospital care were 32.4% of GDP, spending for retirement communities and nursing care facilities were 4.9%, clinical and physician services were 19.9%, and prescription drug expenditures were 9.8% (CDC, 2017a).

Accessibility Costs

According to the US Census Bureau (2019), the uninsured American is usually a male between the ages of 19 and 64; he has a low income and less (26.9%) than a high school education. Approximately, 11.8% of the US population has less than a high school diploma. Uninsured Americans disproportionately reside in the South and are more likely to be employed in service occupations—approximately one in three, with one in five employed in service occupations in the US as a whole. Non-Hispanic Whites represent nearly four in ten of the uninsured, while six in ten in the overall US are non-Hispanic Whites. Ethnic- minorities and non-Whites represent the 39.3% of the uninsured (US Census Bureau, 2019).

Unequal access to health care is a problem that can manifest itself in different ways, but often it is related to a lack of financial means and insufficient community support systems. Vulnerable populations, such as persons with disabilities, those living in poverty or residing in inner-city or rural areas, children and women, older adults, and ethnic minorities have been identified in national trends (ODPHP, 2019) as being at risk for disparities in healthcare. **Social determinants of health** consist of factors related to the social situations and environments within which people are born, live, age, and work (ODPHP, 2019). The social determinants of health care disparities coincide developmentally from birth to death and are affected by the available community-based resources, familial relationships, low-income neighborhoods, joblessness, drug and alcohol use, sexual promiscuity, and the lack of food and transportation.

When people are unable to access health care treatment because of social and environmental factors in their lives, their health is inevitably compromised. An example would be a client diagnosed with diabetes who does not have transportation to a grocery store that sells fresh fruits and vegetables; in many communities, the closest store is 20 miles from their home and requires transportation by a public bus. Another example is a married mother of two children under the age of three who is diagnosed with sickle cell anemia and misses appointments at a hospital-based medical clinic because of her reliance on public transportation and need for childcare. When the accessibility of healthcare facilities is an issue, consistency in receiving care for disease management can be difficult for those affected. Hence, social determinants, such as lack of funds to pay for transportation, lack of access to healthy foods and grocery stores that provide nutritious options, and lack of familial support or neighborhood childcare, can all impact clients' health.

- Socioeconomic Impact on Health

The Poor and Wage Earning

Socioeconomic factors have a significant role in health disparities among all people receiving health care in the US. The ability to pay for services or treat one's disease or illness with medications, dietary interventions, exercise, and mental health counseling or therapy in a safe and clean environment is not easily achievable for all. Statistics from the second quarter of 2019 on the weekly earnings of salary and wage workers in the US noted that the number of full-time workers totaled 117.6 million with a median weekly salary of $908 (Bureau of Labor Statistics, 2019).

Median weekly earnings for salary and wage workers calculated by major ethnic and racial groups indicated the following wage gaps for full-time employed workers: Whites ($933), Hispanics ($696), Asians ($1,152), and Blacks ($724; Bureau of Labor Statistics, 2019). These data were not adjusted for labor that is seasonally affected, such as construction, painting outdoors, or farm work. When there are financial wage gaps, accessibility to health care can be further complicated, with persons being unable to pay for health care as customers, either with or without insurance.

While wage gaps continue to exist, in 2019, according to the US Census Bureau (2020), there was an increase in the median household income for all Americans. An increase of this kind has historically only occurred five times since the US began recording income data in 1959. A 6.8% increase in the income of Asian, Hispanic, Black, and White Americans' incomes occurred in 2019—from $64,324 in 2018 to $68,703 in 2019 (US Census Bureau, 2020).

The Poor and Exposure to Environmental Pollutants

According to Pleasants et al. (2016), chronic obstructive pulmonary disease (COPD) is a global health problem that primarily impacts people of low SES. The poor are disproportionately more likely than their wealthier counterparts to be exposed to environmental pollutants from tobacco, indoor biomass fuel, and occupational inhalation of toxins. Additionally, sociopolitical factors and health behaviors also affect persons of low SES. The World Health Organization (WHO, 2018) estimates that, each year worldwide, 7 million people die as a result of factors related to air pollution; 80% of these people reside in urban areas within low-to middle-income countries. Current WHO (2018) data note that nine out of ten people around the world are exposed to air polluted by industrial facilities; residential lighting that polluting fuels, cooking, and heating; heat and power generation; agricultural and municipal waste burning/incineration and waste sites; and fuel combustion from motor vehicles.

In 2005, 3 million people died from COPD (WHO, 2018). Over 90% of these deaths were within low- or middle-income geographical regions. The Global Initiative for Chronic Lung Disease, a global strategy for the diagnosis, management, and prevention of COPD, in 2018 developed a report on the worldwide impacts of this respiratory disease. The report outlined how COPD should no longer be viewed as a chronic disease process with progressive damage to the human body leading to death, but as a preventable illness.

Pleasants et al. (2016) noted that asthma, a health deviation also experienced by people of low SES, is exacerbated by air pollution as well. They offered recommendations to lower the prevalence of COPD (and asthma) as health disparities in low-SES areas, including decreasing occupational exposure, minimizing biomass fuels, and smoking cessation. Furthermore, they suggested educating health care workers and others involved in the provision of care for persons at risk for developing, or diagnosed with, COPD, and ensuring that affordable health care and improvements in the cost-effective delivery of care are promoted. Improvements in the surveillance of the undiagnosed public and of persons diagnosed with COPD in economically disadvantaged groups can potentially prevent this respiratory disease and decrease its worldwide impact.

Chronic Stress, Illness, and Racial/ Ethnic Minority Research

The chronicity of illness occurs with multiple acute episodes of illness secondary to an ineffective treatment of diseases or conditions. Exposure to stress over long periods of time (Jackson et al., 2010) can result in the development of health problems. Stress has been identified as a factor in the development of mental illnesses, such as anxiety and depression, and physical ailments, such as cancer, asthma, and heart disease. Hence, heightened and prolonged stress may be detrimental to affected persons' health.

Epidemiological studies of racial and ethnic minorities' physical and mental health show evidence of low life expectancy, with mortality and morbidity at the forefront of many illnesses. For example, African American males have statistically higher rates of prostate cancer than do White males (National Institutes of Health [NIH], 2018). In cancer disparity research, it is still unknown why African American men are more likely than other males to develop aggressive forms of prostate cancer. Currently, Black men have a 15% greater chance of being diagnosed with prostate cancer than their White male counterparts, whose probability of such a diagnosis is 10%.

In 2018, the NIH, National Cancer Institute, National Institute on Minority Health and Health Disparities (NIMHD), and the Prostate Cancer Foundation began a collaboratively funded study examining the biological and non-biological factors potentially involved in the development of aggressive prostate cancer in African American males. The study, titled "Research on Prostate Cancer in Men of African Ancestry: Defining the Roles of Genetics, Tumor Markers, and Social Stress (RESPOND)," has a budget of $26.5 million. The goal is to enroll 10,000 African American men who have been diagnosed with prostate cancer. Discrimination, early-life experiences, segregation, and environmental and neighborhood exposures are being explored in addition to genetic studies of gene variants, tumor samples, and deoxyribonucleic acid (NIH, 2018).

In comparison to Americans of European descent, Black Americans have historically had a lower average life expectancy: 76.1 years for Blacks and 79.8 years for Whites (CDC, 2017b; Jackson, 1993; Jackson et al., 2010). Black men, on average, have a lower life expectancy than Black women, with Black men living 72.9 years (69.5 to 71.5) and Black women living 78.9 years (76.4 to 78.1). Similarly, White males have a life expectancy of 77.5 years (75.7 to 76.1), and White females' average life expectancy is 82.0 years (80.6 to 81.0). Finally, Hispanic males' average life expectancy is 79.6 years (77.5 to 79.1), while Hispanic females have an average life expectancy of 84.1 years (82.9 to 84.3; CDC, 2017b; CDC, 2019).

The correlations between stress and health disparities have been attributed to differences in financial stability, race, gender, level of education, residing in rural or inner cities, and marital status (i.e., being married vs. unmarried or widowed). Westby et al. (2016) examined body mass index (BMI), gender, the impact of social support on mental and physical health, and race with regard to health-related quality of life (HRQoL) for cancer survivors. Using two-step multiple linear regressions, a participant group of 1,768 male and female cancer survivors were assessed for mental and physical health quality. The data were obtained from the American Cancer Society's (ACS) cross-sectional Study of Cancer Survivors.

Criteria for eligibility in the Westby et al. (2016) study included being: (1) a resident of a target state at the time of diagnosis; (2) 18-years of age or older at the time of diagnosis; (3) diagnosed in a calendar year two, five, or 10 years prior to sampling; (4) diagnosed with one of the six incident cancer sites of interest; and (5) diagnosed with local, regional, or distant Surveillance, Epidemiology, and End Results (SEER; cancer statistics) summary stage cancer (including in situ bladder cancer cases). The six incident cancer sites identified in the study were melanoma, uterine, bladder, prostate, breast, and colorectal cancers (Westby et al., 2016, p. 411). The average age of participants was 67.4 years, and the majority of the participants were non-Hispanic Whites (85.9%, n = 1,517), in a marriage-like relationship (69.7%, n = 1,232), and female (53.3%, n = 941). Participants' self-reported BMI was 28.33 with a standard deviation of 5.90; 729 (41.3%) participants reported being overweight, and 535 (30.3%) participants reported being obese.

Exclusionary criteria for the Westby et al. (2016) study were illness, an inability to communicate in Spanish or English, and mental incompetence. A total of 36,372 cancer survivors were included in the sampled population, and 26,802 survivors were contacted once consent was obtained from their health care providers. Ultimately, 9,105 cancer survivors consented to participate in the study. With HRQoL as the focus of the research, the final sample size became 1,767.

Of interest were the identified comorbidities of study participants. Reported health deviations of hypertension, cardiac problems, diabetes, COPD, emphysema, arthritis, and asthma were noted among a participant group that was described as being impacted by cancer-related factors, social support, physical and mental HRQoL, BMI, and sociodemographics. The latter factors had racial and gender implications. This study is reflective of the distinctive variations in healthcare and outcomes that correlate with low-income status and race.

The Office of Minority Health Research, founded in 1990, is located at the NIH in Bethesda, Maryland. In 2000, the office was elevated by the US government to the Center of Minority Health Research (Perez-Stable & Rodriguez, 2019). It was renamed to NIMHD when the **Patient Protection and Affordable Care Act (ACA)** was enacted in 2010. The ACA is a comprehensive health care reform law that has three targeted goals: (1) to make health insurance affordable and accessible to all Americans by providing subsidies to consumers via tax credits, with the goal of targeting households with incomes that are between 100% and 400% of the federal poverty level in order to cover lower-priced insurance policies; (2) to extend the Medicaid program to cover the insurance needs of Americans with incomes below 138% of the federal poverty level; and (3) to support new and innovative healthcare delivery methodologies that are designed to lower medical costs (Healthcare.gov, n.d.).

With the mission of improving the health of racial and ethnic minorities in the US, the NIMHD began to develop research studies that examined health disparities affecting Native Americans and Alaskan Natives, Asians, Native Hawaiians and other Pacific Islanders, Latinx communities, and African Americans (Perez-Stable & Rodriguez, 2019). In the US, ethnicity, race, and gender are predictors of life expectancy. Additionally, persons with household incomes below the **federal poverty level** have a mortality rate three times that of persons with a higher income (e.g., $115,000). In 2021, a single person residing within the 48 contiguous states or the District of Columbia with an annual income of $12,880 would fall below the federal poverty level; for single residents of Alaska and Hawaii, the corresponding income levels are $16,090 and $14,820, respectively (US DHHS, 2021).

There remains a deficit of racial and ethnic diversity in the healthcare workforce, as well as the biomedical scientific and clinical workforces. Hence, the shortages of diversity in these fields impacts the likelihood of research being completed on minority populations. In 2017, a survey was conducted by the Forum of State Nursing Workforce Centers and the National Council of State Boards of Nursing. The results of the survey were that within the profession of nursing, 7.5% of nurses were Asian, 6.2% were African American, 0.4% were American Indian/Native Alaskan, 5.3%, 2.9% other nurses, 0.5% were Native Hawaiian/Pacific Islander, 80.8% were White/Caucasian, and 1.7% were of two or more races (American Association of Colleges of Nursing, 2019). In 2018, according to the American Association of Medical Colleges (AAMC), 17.1% of physicians were Asian, 5.8% were Hispanic, 5.0% were Black or African American, and 56.2% were White (AAMC, 2021).

Statistically speaking, diversity equates to equity. Unfortunately, racism and discrimination remain a part of US society. The Kaiser Family Foundation conducted a survey asking Americans whether or not they had experienced any discrimination within the last 30 days because of their ethnicity or race. the results showed that 15% of Whites, 36% of Latinx, and 53% of African Americans reported unfair treatment (DiJulio et al., 2019). Discrimination and racism impact all Americans and can contribute to mental and physical stress, which ultimately manifests as illness and disease.

SUMMARY

Health disparities are complex and, at times, difficult to recognize, quantify, and evaluate. However, the data demonstrating the differences that society dictates for persons of low-income and racial and ethnic minorities provide evidence that there is a worldwide problem in the ways that human beings interact, live, and value one another. Access to health care is shrouded with the complexities of cost, availability, environmental safety, and the devaluing of those deemed different or less fortunate in life.

Figure 1. Health disparities isolate and weigh us down

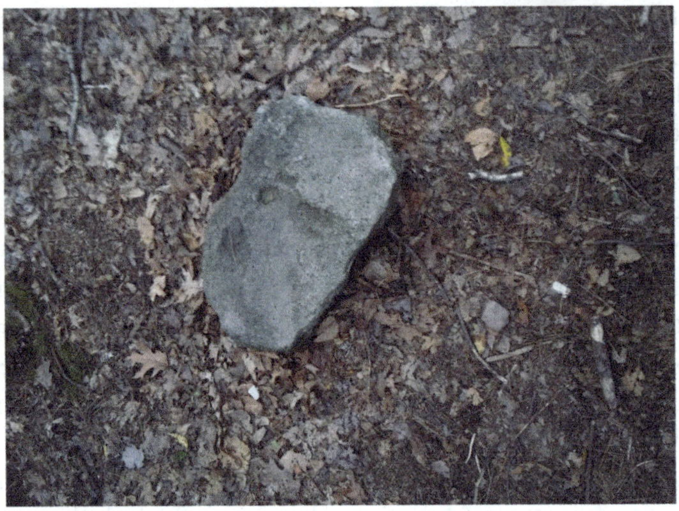

SELF-EXPLORATION AND CONTEMPLATION

Directions: The purpose of self-exploration and contemplation is to encourage innovation and creativity that has, at its foundation, a genuine care and desire to improve one's situation in life and that of others. Self-exploration and contemplation can only occur when a sufficient amount of knowledge and awareness has been attained. Hence, it is with newfound knowledge that personal change can occur, and the adaptation of these changes into our own lives and the lives of others can lead to further growth.

After reading each statement and question, consider how you can personally implement changes that can impact health disparities in your geographical area and improve your own health outcomes as well as those of others.

Consider This

1. Why is it important that all Americans receive quality evidenced-based health care?
2. Does learning about health inequities and disparities impact how you interact with your health care provider? If yes, in what ways?
3. Whose responsibility is it to address health disparities and inequities?
4. Should health disparities and inequities encountered by individuals be addressed by the government at the state or local levels? What about the federal level?
5. Why do health disparities exist, and is it my responsibility as a member of society to care and respond to this issue?
6. Are health disparities and inequities a public health problem?
7. Are financial circumstances or socioeconomic factors in health disparities an issue for all people accessing health care?
8. Do language barriers impact healthcare access and adequacy of care delivery?
9. Are health care disparities and inequities a new problem nationally?
10. Can discrimination be a factor in determining who receives quality and safe evidence-based health care?
11. Is it necessary for healthcare organizations to have diversity in their workforce?
12. Why should the American people care that there are shortages of persons of diverse backgrounds delivering health care (i.e., physicians and nurses) in the US? How does this impact health disparities?

HEALTHCARE AFFORDABILITY: WHO IS GOING TO PAY FOR THIS?

Directions: Health care is expensive. Taxes can vary in amount based on your geographical location. When considering enactments of laws, such as the Affordable Care Act, should all Americans be required to have health insurance? If all Americans are working and can contribute financially to maintaining health insurance coverage, should those working carry the financial responsibility?

1. How does health care inequity impact persons of low income, the working poor, and the underinsured?
2. Should all Americans have access to affordable health care, even if they are not participating in the workforce?
3. Is health care a burden or a privilege?

CASE STUDY: "I COULD NOT AFFORD IT"

The lived experience of a client's voice: I work the overnight shift at an industrial factory making parts. I've done this type of work for 15 years. My dad did it for 35 years, so I guess you can say I kept it in the family. It's a good honest living; the hours just aren't that great. I eat breakfast at 8:00 a.m. when I get home; then I go straight to bed. My wife and the kids clear out of the house quickly. I kiss them goodbye and I sleep until about 8:00 p.m. I go back to work again at midnight. I am 55 years old. I used to get up at 8:00 p.m. and exercise, but now my activity level has changed.

About eight months ago, during my annual physical, my doctor pointed out that I had gained about 15 pounds too much. My hemoglobin A1C was 8 mg/dL, and my fasting blood glucose was 299 mg/dL. I had diabetes. I was prescribed Metformin, but my blood sugar was still high. I lost weight and was thirsty a lot. The doctor put me on Humulin R and Humulin N insulin. I have two kids in college. When the tuition for both of my son's schools went up, I decided to briefly not purchase my insulin, and went for one month without my medication. The medication cost too much and I could not afford it. I got sick and ended up in the hospital.

I work hard for my family. I have health insurance, but it covers the bare minimum. I have a good job, do the best I can, and I still do not have enough money to get my health needs taken care of . . . it's hard. I do not know what I can do. I am too proud to ask anyone for help. Who does that? I'll just have to try and get a second job.

Discussion: Are there currently any financial resources outside of the monies from the private insurance available that could be offered to this gentleman to ensure that he is able to purchase his insulin?

REFERENCES

American Association of Colleges of Nursing. (2019). *Enhancing diversity in the workforce*. https://www.aacnnursing.org/News-Information/Fact-Sheets/Enhancing-Diversity

Association of American Medical Colleges. (2021). *Figure 18. Percentage of all active physicians by race/ethnicity, 2018*. https://www.aamc.org/data-reports/workforce/interactive-data/figure-18-percentage-all-active-physicians-race/ethnicity-2018

Bureau of Labor Statistics. (2019, July 17). *Usual weekly earnings of wage and salary workers, second quarter 2019*. https://www.bls.gov/news.release/pdf/wkyeng.pdf

Centers for Disease Control and Prevention. (2017a). *National Center for Health Statistics: Health expenditures*. https://www.cdc.gov/nchs/fastats/health-expenditures.htm

Centers for Disease Control and Prevention. (2017b). *Summary health statistics: National Health Interview Survey*. https://minorityhealth.hhs.gov/omh/browse.aspx?lvl=4&lvlid=75

Centers for Disease Control and Prevention. (2019). *National Vital Statistics Report: United States life tables, 2017*. https://www.cdc.gov/nchs/data/nvsr/nvsr68/nvsr68_07-508.pdf

Colby, S. L., & Ortman, J. M. (2015). *Projections of the size and composition of the U.S. Population: 2014 to 2060*. U.S. Census Bureau. https://www.census.gov/content/dam/Census/library/publications/2015/demo/p25-1143.pdf

DiJulio, B., Norton, M., Jackson, S., & Brodie, M. (2015). *Kaiser Family Foundation/CNN survey of Americans on race*. Kaiser Family Foundation. https://files.kff.org/attachment/report-survey-of-americans-on-race

Global Initiative for Chronic Obstructive Lung Disease. (2018). *Global strategy for diagnosis, Management, and prevention of chronic obstructive pulmonary disease*. https://goldcopd.org/wp-content/uploads/2018/11/GOLD-2019-v1.7-FINAL-14Nov2018-WMS.pdf

Harvard, T. H. Chan School of Public Health. (2008). *Julius Richmond, former U.S. Surgeon General and Professor of Health Policy, Emeritus, dies.* https://www.hsph.harvard.edu/news/press-releases/julius-richmond-former-us-surgeon-general-dies/

Health Equity Institute. (2019). *Defining health equity*. https://healthequity.sfsu.edu/content/defining-health-equity

HealthCare.gov. (n.d.). *Affordable Care Act (ACA)*. https://www.healthcare.gov/glossary/affordable-care-act/

Jackson, J. S. (1993). African American experiences through the adult years. In The encyclopedia of adult development (pp. 18–26). Oryx Press.

Jackson, J. S., Knight, K. M., & Rafferty, J. A. (2010). Race and unhealthy behaviors: Chronic stress, the HPA Axis, and physical and mental health disparities over the life course. *American Journal of Public Health*, *100*(5), 933–939. doi:10.2105/AJPH.2008.143446 PMID:19846689

National Institutes of Health. (2018). *NIH and Prostate Cancer Foundation launch large study on aggressive prostate cancer in African American men*. https://www.nih.gov/news-events/news-releases/nih-prostate-cancer-foundation-launch-large-study-aggressive-prostate-cancer-AfricanAmerican-men launch-large-study-aggressive-prostate-cancer-African American-men

Office of Disease Prevention and Health Promotion. (2019). *Healthy People 2020*. Retrieved on July 5, 2019, from https://www.healthypeople.gov/

Office of Disease Prevention and Health Promotion. (2021). *Healthy People 2030*. Retrieved on March 30, 2021, from https://www.healthypeople.gov/

Parker, K., Horowitz, J. M., Brown, A., Fry, R., Cohn, D., & Igielnik, R. (2018). Demographic and economic trends in urban, suburban and rural communities. *Pew Research*. https://www.pewresearch.org/social-trends/2018/05/22/demographic-and-economic-trends-in-urban-suburban-and-rural-communities/

Perez-Stable, E. J., & Rodriguez, E. J. (2019). Uniting the vision for health equity through partnerships: The 2nd annual Dr. Elijah Saunders & Dr. Levi Watkins Memorial Lecture. *Ethnicity & Disease*, *29*(Suppl 1), 193–200. doi:10.18865/ed.29.S1.193 PMID:30906169

Physicians for a National Health Program. (2019). *Influence watch*. https://www.influencewatch.org/non-profit/physicians-for-a-national-health-program-pnhp/

Pleasants, R. A., Riley, I. L., & Mannino, D. M. (2016). Defining and targeting health disparities in chronic obstructive pulmonary disease. *International Journal of Chronic Pulmonary Obstructive Disease*, *11*, 2475–2496. doi:10.2147/COPD.S79077 PMID:27785005

United States Census Bureau. (2019). *Who are the uninsured? Most uninsured were working-age adults*. https://www.census.gov/library/stories/2018/09/who-are-the-uninsured.html

United States Department of Health & Human Services. (2021). *Office of the Assistant Secretary for Planning and Evaluation: Poverty guidelines*. https://aspe.hhs.gov/poverty-guidelines

Vespa, J., Medina, L., & Armstrong, D. M. (2020). *Demographic turning points for the United States: Population projections for 2020 to 2060*. U.S. Census Bureau. https://www.census.gov/content/dam/Census/library/publications/2020/demo/p25-1144.pdf

Westby, R., Berg, C., & Leach, C. (2016). Gender, race, BMI, and social support in relation to the health-related quality of life of cancer survivors: A report from the American Cancer Society's Study of Cancer Survivors II (SCS-II). *Quality of Life Research: An International Journal of Quality of Life Aspects of Treatment, Care and Rehabilitation*, *25*(2), 409–421. doi:10.100711136-015-1084-6 PMID:26289021

World Health Organization. (2018). *Air pollution*. https://www.who.int/health-topics/air-pollution#tab=tab_1

Chapter 2
Historical Overview of Health Disparities in the United States

ABSTRACT

Health disparities in the United States and around the world carry with them a history of cultural bias, fear of the unknown, racism, sexism, ageism, intolerance of religious beliefs, and a desire to retain the status quo. Some people perceive a majority group as superior to demographic groups that are believed to be inferior. However, as the US population becomes increasingly diverse, changes will come. Internationally, globalization and immigration merge the worlds of the poor and rich, as each social class struggles to find their socioeconomic and healthcare footprint in modern-day society. All US citizens will be affected by a failure to unite.

LEARNING OBJECTIVES

1. Explain why Jews were persecuted by the Third Reich Nazi regime during the years 1933–1945.
2. Determine the medical necessity and indications for the Tuskegee Syphilis Research Study for African American men.
3. Discuss whether or not it was morally correct to not inform the living biological relatives of Mrs. Henrietta Lacks of the medical research community's postmortem use of her cervical cellular tissue.

DOI: 10.4018/978-1-7998-3874-6.ch002

4. Describe what occurred within the Willowbrook healthcare facility and consider whether facilities like this currently exist. Are adults and children still abused in long-term treatment facilities?
5. Explain the importance of informed consent in the Jewish Chronic Disease Hospital Study.

Reflection Quote: "It seems incomprehensible that human beings can consciously choose to do harm to one another."

INTRODUCTION

The idea of a modern society that has innovative medicine and advanced surgical procedures having to use the terminology "health disparities" seems an oxymoron. However, among low-income people and racial and ethnic minorities, health disparities are faced on a regular basis, including each time they interface with healthcare systems. People's lifespans are impacted by their demographic group and geographical location.

The narratives of the poor as well as religious, racial, and ethnic minorities within the US and abroad have been associated with discriminatory practices in health care. Rather than being valued, people's differences are often perceived as unacceptable. By minimizing the value of a human life, we subject those affected to self-hatred, isolation, feelings of unwontedness, and not belonging. This chapter explores the physical and emotional harm that humans have bestowed upon others they have deemed different and worthless. It is important to note that anyone can be treated wrongfully. Targets of maltreatment are often perceived by others as a threat to their societal presence and impact, or as a disruption to the status quo.

UNETHICAL MEDICAL EXPERIMENTATION

The Nazis and the Holocaust

In Europe, for the promotion of what was deemed a **pure race**, members of the Third Reich Nazi regime (1933–1945) performed unethical medical experiments on Jewish people whom the Nazis had imprisoned in concentration camps. The medical experiments included exposure to poisons, freezing temperatures, high altitudes, malaria, untested drugs, and typhus. Euthanasia, sterilization, and surgical procedures without the use of anesthesia were also performed (Berger, 1990; Steinfels & Levine, 1976; Weindling, 2005).

These unethical experiments performed on Jews, as well as their intentional gassing in chambers within concentration camps and other atrocities, were mandated solely for the purpose of murdering innocent Jewish men, women, and children. Estimates of the number of Jewish people killed during this mass genocide, known as **the Holocaust**, have varied from 4.8 million to 6.2 million (Bard, 2021). There is no logical reason for the occurrence of these atrocities, and the Holocaust and Nazi persecution serve as a reminder of the depths of depravity to which humans will go to eliminate or harm those they deem to be different.

US Public Health Service Research

African American men residing in the rural town of Tuskegee, Alabama, in 1932 were made the subjects of a study on syphilis by the US Public Health Service (Rothman, 1982). **Syphilis** is a sexually transmitted infection that is bacterial in origin and caused by *Treponema pallidum*. The infection is spread through sexual contact and from mother to fetus, and to the infant during the birthing process (CDC, 2021). *Treponema pallidum* are spirochetes that enter the mucous membranes of the genitalia and mouth. Syphilis infection is spread as a result of the entry of these spirochetes and manifests as a chancre—a round firm ulcer that has the spirochetes inside it. Syphilis is highly contagious.

With the initial infection of syphilis, infected persons can develop symptoms, on average, approximately 21 days (or 10–90 days) after contagion. While a chancre can last for three to six weeks, syphilis remains active in the body. Untreated syphilis progresses from the primary stage of the infection to the secondary and tertiary stages.

African American men who were diagnosed with syphilis were observed by healthcare providers and workers participating in the Tuskegee syphilis research study. Intentionally left untreated, the men likely experienced all three stages of syphilis because the infection can last for several decades. Syphilis, therefore, is both an acute and chronic disease. The following are the three stages of syphilis:

1. **Primary Syphilis:** Presents two to three weeks post-infection as a painless lesion, the chancre. The chancre resolves on its own in 3–12 weeks without any treatment.
2. **Secondary Syphilis:** The infection is no longer localized as it was in presentation with the chancre; it is now generalized. Infected persons have a rash that can last from one week to six months; the rash covers the soles of the feet, the neck to the pelvis area, the arms and legs, and the palms of the hands. Additionally, patients can experience fever, weight loss, arthritis, meningitis, malaise, hair loss, and swollen lymph nodes. Contagion with the presence of lesion(s) remains. A **latency stage** follows the secondary stage whereby the infected person has no symptoms; however, symptoms of secondary syphilis return.
3. **Tertiary Syphilis:** The third stage is a slow and progressive inflammatory process whereby multiple organs of the body are affected. Patients can experience meningitis, stroke, psychosis, dementia, or paresis as a result of aortitis (inflammation of the aortic wall) and neurosyphilis (Grossman & Porth, 2014; Hinkle & Cheever, 2018).

The African American men who participated in the study were not provided education on the purpose of the study or the implications of the research in which they were involved. Some of the men were unaware that they were even a part of a research study. The purpose of the study was to examine how syphilis, untreated, affected African American men. There was a control group and a group of men known to researchers to be experiencing active signs and symptoms of syphilis infection.

Four years into the study, in 1936, African American men who had syphilis began to develop health complications. Although examined periodically by the researchers, the affected men were never treated even though the antibiotic penicillin was identified as an effective treatment for syphilis in the 1940s.

Researchers from the US Public Health Service Tuskegee Syphilis Study began disseminating their findings through publications in 1936 and every four to six years thereafter. No one in the government or private sector attempted to stop the study. The study continued and received the support of the CDC in 1969 (Brandt, 1978; Rothman, 1982). The *Washington Star* (also known as the *Washington Star-News* and the *Washington Evening Star*), a newspaper that was published daily in Washington, DC, from 1852 until 1981 (DC Public Library, 2020), published an article in 1972 that explained how the syphilis study was implemented and continued to affect the African

American participants. After the story ran, the Tuskegee Syphilis Study was investigated, deemed unethical, and stopped.

Institutional Research on Disabled Children

The Willowbrook State Developmental Center, an institution located in Staten Island, New York, provided services to adults and children with disabilities. The Willowbrook facility was comprised of a group of buildings known to have had as many as 6,200 residents in 1969, when it was meant to accommodate only 4,000. Willowbrook was not only overcrowded, but also reportedly understaffed; residents were unkempt and the housing facilities were unclean (Disability Justice, 2020; Rothman, 1982).

Between the mid-1950s and early 1970s, Dr. Saul Krugman, a physician, conducted research on children residing at Willowbrook. The children were intentionally infected with the hepatitis virus. The rationale for the study was that the children would likely become infected with hepatitis at Willowbrook because they would be adapting to institutional living. Admissions to the facility were contingent on the children's parents granting permission for their children to join the study and be injected with the hepatitis virus. The benefits of the study were touted as the children receiving more direct staff care, clinical oversight, and cleaner environments in which to live (Rothman, 1982).

The Willowbrook study lasted approximately 20 years. Dr. Krugman and his associates published several research articles describing their findings and protocols. Beecher (1966) noted in an article published in the *New England Journal of Medicine* that the Willowbrook study was unethical. However, the virus injections continued for the facility's residents until the early 1970s. Willowbrook was opened in 1942 and finally closed its doors in 1987 (Disability Justice, 2020).

Absence of Informed Consent

In 1962, Dr. Chester Southam, a physician practicing at the Sloan-Kettering Institute for Cancer Research, was granted permission by the Jewish Chronic Disease Hospital in Brooklyn, New York, to conduct a cancer study. The proposed purpose of the study was to determine if patients that were compromised by cancer could reject live cancer cells injected into their bodies. Twenty-two patients participated in the study (Hershey & Miller, 1976; Levine, 1986).

Informed consent is when patients are provided information about treatment options and surgical procedures, and their associated risks and benefits (Hinkle & Cheever, 2018). Dr. Southam and his colleagues did not inform the 22 study participants that the injections administered to them were live cancer cells. Once it was determined that the patients did not receive information about the risks and benefits of the study (i.e., that no informed consent was provided), the study was terminated (Azuine & Ekejiuba, 2015).

HeLa Cells

Mrs. Henrietta Lacks, a married African American mother of five children, presented to Johns Hopkins Hospital in Baltimore, Maryland, in 1951. The 31-year-old had been experiencing vaginal bleeding. the physician who saw her, Dr. Howard Jones, upon completion of a vaginal examination, diagnosed Mrs. Lack with cervical cancer. After receiving this diagnosis, Mrs. Lacks was prescribed radium treatments.

A renowned virus and cancer researcher, Dr. George Gey, obtained Mrs. Lacks' s cervical tissue, which had been retrieved during a biopsy procedure. Reportedly, Dr. Gey had samples of other patients' cervical tissue, which he maintained in the lab, but the tissue samples would die in short periods of time. However, Mrs. Lacks's tissue cells doubled every 20 to 24 hours. The rapid productivity and viability of Mrs. Lacks's cells was an extraordinary scientific finding (Johns Hopkins Medicine, 2021).

Mrs. Lacks succumbed to cervical cancer on October 4, 1951. Her cellular tissue was used without her permission, nor that of her family. In the 1950s, Johns Hopkins Hospital was atypical in that they granted care to African Americans; many hospitals would refuse to care for low-income Black patients. Hence, the care that was offered was less likely to be challenged or questioned by minorities who were provided access to health care and potential cures of diseases (Johns Hopkins Medicine, 2021).

It was not until the 1970s that Mrs. Lacks's biological family discovered that their deceased family member's cellular tissue was being used to study the effects of viruses, hormones, and drugs on the growth of cancer cells in lieu of human experimentation. The Lacks family was contacted by a scientist seeking to obtain genetic materials and blood samples from Henrietta's descendants. In 1998, a documentary developed by the British Broadcasting

Corporation told the story of the unethical global distribution of the genetic material in the absence of the Lacks family's permission (consent). Author Rebecca Skloot wrote a book further detailing Mrs. Lacks's life and the unethical use of her cells, titled *The Immortal Life of Henrietta Lacks*. Mrs. Lacks's cellular tissue, now referred to as **HeLa Cells**, has been used worldwide and sold to researchers. The Lacks family now receives credit in scientific research papers that have used their genetic material (Biography, 2021; Johns Hopkins Medicine, 2021).

ADDRESSING THE HISTORICAL DANGERS OF HUMAN SUBJECTS RESEARCH

Two years after the end of the Second World War, 16 German physicians were convicted of the crimes they committed against the Jews and other persons they imprisoned and on whom they conducted unethical medical research. In 1947, the Nuremberg Code, a set of guidelines for research, was developed to ensure that medical studies involving human subjects were ethically sound, conducted humanely, and involved consent on the part of participants. In 1964, the Declaration of Helsinki reiterated the importance of informed consent in research, and in 1978, the Belmont Report emphasized the principles of justice, respect for persons, and beneficence in all research endeavors, especially those involving human subjects (Constantin, 2018).

Federal regulations for the protection of human subjects were developed by the US Department of Health and Human Services (US DHHS) in 1981 and revised as needed over the years. The Code of Federal Regulations (CFR), Title 45, Part 46, Protection of Human Subjects, developed in 2009, reinforced the documentation of informed consent, the use of an institutional review board (IRB) to review all proposed research materials for ethical processes, and the protection of all human subjects, including additional protections specifically for prisoners, neonates, children, human fetuses, and pregnant woman (US DHHS, 2010). Revisions in 2018 to CFR Title 45, Part 46, were made to the IRB requirements in Section 46.109 (f) (1) (i) and to Section 12 of the Newborn Screening Saves Lives Reauthorization Act of 2014 (the Common Rule), which regulates the use of newborn dried blood spots in research (US DHHS, 2019).

The US Food and Drug Administration (FDA) and the US DHHS provide regulations for both behavioral and biomedical research. The FDA has its own regulations to ensure the protection of human subjects during clinical investigations involving drugs, cosmetics, and food. Further protection of the public's health information was initiated in 2003 via Public Law 104-191, the Health Insurance Portability and Accountability Act (commonly referred to as HIPAA).

Healthcare workers and providers are responsible for the delivery of care to patients based upon their presenting diagnosis and immediate health deviations. From an ethical perspective, healthcare workers and providers must demonstrate behaviors toward patients that are morally acceptable. Ross (1930/2002) coined the phrase *prima facie duties*, which refers to a duty to self. The duties to oneself encompass the promotion of good on the behalf of others, ensuring that others are treated equally, and the avoidance of doing wrong to others.

Ross's (1930/2002) *prima facie duties* include:

- Nonmaleficence (no injury to others),
- Fidelity (keep promises),
- Beneficence (improve the condition of others),
- Gratitude (thank those that help),
- Justice (recognition of merit),
- Reparation (compensate others when harm is done to them), and
- Self-improvement (improvement of intelligence and virtue).

Unfortunately, while research studies have guidelines that have been substantiated and upheld in courts of law after clear violations of the rights of human subjects, unethical practices can still occur in healthcare-associated research. While governments have developed federal regulations to protect human subjects, the poor, illiterate, and racial and ethnic minorities can still fall prey to injustices occurring in modern-day healthcare facilities. These injustices can manifest as violations of duty ethics by healthcare workers and providers. However, today's unethical practices can be more covert, manifesting themselves under the terminology of *health disparities*.

HEALTH DISPARITIES

Health disparities are opportunities to achieve optimal health through preventable means with regard to injury, burden of disease, and violence, that are thwarted because a person(s) comes from a socially disadvantaged group

(CDC, 2008, 2018). Education, geographic location, income, ethnicity, sexual orientation, disability, race, gender, and religion are all factors attributed to inequities that disadvantaged groups experience because of who they are or are perceived to represent. Because of their differences, others—both consciously and unconsciously—deem them unworthy recipients of high-quality, evidenced-based health care.

SUMMARY

Historically, disadvantaged groups classified and identified by the labeling of society have been denied quality health care. Unethical experimentations, physical and emotional abuse, and denial of treatment have been the hallmarks of persons experiencing health disparities worldwide. Healthcare workers and providers are obligated ethically, as licensed professionals providing services to the public, to treat others who are different from themselves with respect, integrity, and care, and to ensure that all people receive quality health care in a timely manner that is evidenced-based and promotes optimal health.

DARK WATERS

Directions: Metaphorically, dark waters are places where the depth of the water is unknown. In the darkness lurks danger and trepidation. Unfortunately, when dark waters have a history of death and destruction, fear exists and, subjectively, people tread lightly for fear of being engulfed.

The unethical experiments that have been performed on human beings are a part of society's history of delving into dark waters in absence of care for others as well as accountability. Inhumane behavior is propagated among the living when the value of other beings is perceived to have no worth. Review these questions and statements and consider how, when, and why you will exit dark waters.

1. I believe that my race and culture is superior to others. Explain and validate this statement.
2. Fear can interfere with or thwart logical reasoning. Is this a true or false statement?
3. Scientific experiments involving racial and ethnic-minorities, persons of a different faith, the mentally ill, the disabled, and the poor should

always be under the scrutiny of sponsors of the study, as well as local and federal governments. Should this statement be true—yes or no? Explain why.

4. Do you believe or deny that discrimination no longer exists in modern-day society?
5. What regulations and laws exist to protect human beings from being subjected to unethical scientific or medical experiments?
6. Is it possible that the Tuskegee Syphilis Study could have impacted African Americans' trust of researchers and healthcare providers?
7. Are the rights of disabled people since the Willowbrook Hepatitis Study better protected in the US?
8. Are differences in age, physical appearance, sex, gender, religion, cultural background, language, or skin color factors in how a human being is treated in modern-day society?
9. Have you ever made a personal judgment about someone based on their height or weight?
10. Does a person's skin color or biological differences in nose or lip shape and hair texture coincide with intelligence?

Figure 1. Dark waters

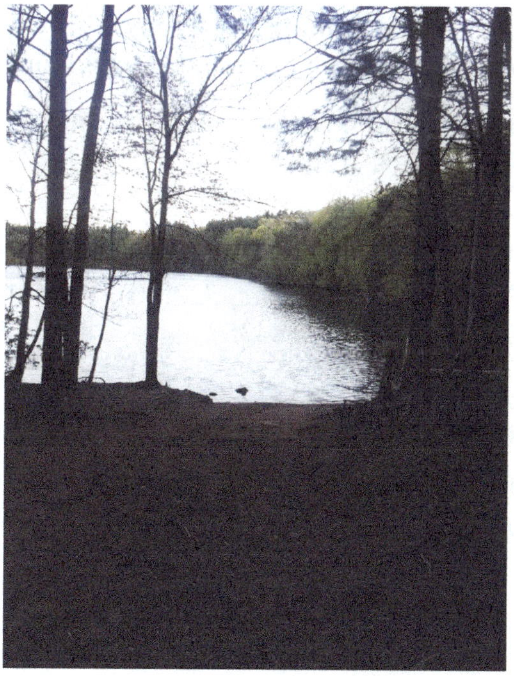

CASE STUDY: NOT INFORMED

The lived experience of a client's voice: When the doctor told me that my son's right arm had an impairment in circulation after he landed on it when he had an accident while riding his motorcycle, I thought that meant that the doctor would fix the circulation problem. I asked him three times, could my son's right arm be saved? The doctor said that she would fix the problem and for me to relax and rejoin my family. Three hours later, my son woke up with a right arm that had been amputated. I signed a form for a doctor to mutilate my son.

Discussion: Should this mother have been updated by the physician during the surgery about the inability to restore circulation to her son's right arm, which potentially led to the unplanned amputation?

REFERENCES

Azuine, R. E., & Ekejiuba, S. E. (2015). Overcoming Challenges in Conducting Clinical Trials in Minority Populations: Identifying and Testing What Works. *International Journal of Maternal Child Health and AIDS, 3*(1), 81–84.

Bard, M. (2021). *Documenting numbers of victims of Holocaust & Nazi persecution.* Jewish Virtual Library (A Project of AICE). https://www.jewishvirtuallibrary.org/documenting-numbers-of-victims-of-the-holocaust

Beecher, H. K. (1966). Ethics and clinical research. *The New England Journal of Medicine, 274*(24), 1354–1360. doi:10.1056/NEJM196606162742405 PMID:5327352

Berger, R. L. (1990). Nazi science: The Dachau hypothermia experiments. *The New England Journal of Medicine, 322*(20), 1435–1440. doi:10.1056/NEJM199005173222006 PMID:2184357

Biography. (2021). *Henrietta Lacks (1920–1951).* https://www.biography.com/scientist/henrietta-lacks

Brandt, A. M. (1978). Racism and research: The case of Tuskegee syphilis study. *The Hastings Center Report, 8*(6), 21–29. doi:10.2307/3561468 PMID:721302

Centers for Disease Control and Prevention. (2008). *Community Health and Program Services (CHAPS): Health disparities among racial/ethnic populations*. United States Department of Health and Human Services.

Centers for Disease Control and Prevention. (2018). *Adolescent and school health: health disparities*. https://www.cdc.gov/healthyyouth/disparities/index.htm

Centers for Disease Control and Prevention. (2021). *Sexually Transmitted Diseases (STD): Syphilis*. https://www.cdc.gov/std/syphilis/default.htm

Constantin, A. (2018). Human subject research: International and regional human rights standards. *Health and Human Rights Journal, 20*(2), 137–148. https://www.ncbi.nlm.nih.gov/pmc/articles/PMC6293356/

D.C. Public Library. (2020). *Washington Evening Star 1852–1981*. https://www.dclibrary.org/eveningstar

Disability Justice. (2020). *The closing of Willowbrook:* New York State Association for Retarded Children v. Carey. https://disabilityjustice.org/the-closing-of-willowbrook/

Grossman, S. C., & Porth, C. M. (2014). *Pathophysiology: Concepts of altered health states* (9th ed.). Lippincott Williams & Wilkins.

Hershey, G. A., & Miller, R. (1976). *Human experimentation and the law*.

Hinkle, J. L., & Cheever, K. H. (2018). *Brunner & Suddarth's textbook of medical-surgical nursing* (14th ed.). Wolters Kluwer.

Johns Hopkins Medicine. (2021). *The legacy of Henrietta Lacks*. https://www.hopkinsmedicine.org/henriettalacks/

Levine, R. J. (1986). *Ethics and regulation of clinical research* (2nd ed.). Urban & Schwarzenberg.

Ross, W. D. (2002). *The right and the good*. Oxford University Press. (Original work published 1930) doi:10.1093/0199252653.001.0001

Rothman, D. J. (1982). Were Tuskegee and Willowbrook "studies in nature?". *The Hastings Center Report, 12*(2), 5–7. doi:10.2307/3561798 PMID:7096065

Steinfels, P., & Levine, C. (1976). Biomedical ethics and the shadow of Nazism. *Hastings Center Report, 614*, 1–20. doi:10.2307/3560386

United States Department of Health and Human Services, Office of Human Research Protections. (2019). *Revised Common Rule Regulatory Text (July 19, 2018).* https://www.hhs.gov/ohrp/regulations-and-policy/regulations/revised-common-rule-regulatory-text/index.html

United States Department of Health and Human Services, Office of Human Research Protections. (201p). *Pre-2018 Requirements (July 14, 2009).* https://www.hhs.gov/ohrp/regulations-and-policy/regulations/regulatory-text/index.html

Weindling, P. (2005). Medicine & the Nuremberg Trials: From medical war crimes to informed consent. *British Medical Journal, 331*(7513), 408. doi:10.1136/bmj.331.7513.408

Chapter 3
Culture, Race, and Ethnicity

ABSTRACT

Race and culture are uniquely different descriptions of all people. Physical characteristics, genetic variations, and geographic location(s) versus the traditions, faiths, and belief systems with which human beings are brought up position each person to view and experience the world and their immediate environments differently. Hence, when people of different races and cultural backgrounds enter the healthcare system, a cultural clash can occur. Evidence of this cultural clash can be manifested, for example, in language barriers, health literacy, and dietary and medication adherence issues. Healthcare workers and providers working collaboratively with professionals in the community can positively enhance the care that affected persons and their families receive, thus breaking the health disparity cycle.

LEARNING OBJECTIVES

1. Compare and contrast differences between the terms *culture* and *race*.
2. Describe how cultural assimilation can affect racial and ethnic minorities' in-group identity.
3. Explain how environmental pollutants and stress can contribute to asthma exacerbations.
4. Describe the role of the school nurse in educating staff and parents about asthma management.

DOI: 10.4018/978-1-7998-3874-6.ch003

Reflection Quote: "Independent of race, anyone can embrace and participate within a culture through marriage, friendship, and faith."

INTRODUCTION

Defining Culture

The National Institutes of Health (NIH, 2021b) describes **culture** as the

> *combination of a body of knowledge, a body of belief, and a body of behavior. It involves several elements that are often specific to ethnic, racial, religious, geographic, or social groups. This includes personal identification, language, thoughts, communications, actions, customs, beliefs, values, and institutions. For the provider of health information or health care, these elements influence belief systems surrounding health, healing, wellness, illness, disease, and delivery of health services.*

Culture encompasses values that are generationally shared by families both in writing and through informal storytelling. Linguistically, culture incorporates language and communication patterns that are unique to communities of people. Culture impacts responses to life events, such as death, celebrations of births, religious events and holidays, pain, and crises.

Subcultures are groups of people who are members of a larger cultural group. Members of a subculture may vary in their physical appearance and occupation compared to the primary culture. Cultural characteristics, such as physical appearance and **ethnicity** (a common heritage, identification) as well as occupation, change when **cultural assimilation** occurs among members of the identified minority culture when they choose to identify with the dominant culture in order to avoid discrimination (Taylor et al., 2019).

Race

Race is typically equated with physical characteristics associated with facial structure and features, skin pigmentation, hair texture, and body stature. The US federal government currently recognizes the following groups as racial groups: White, Native Hawaiian or other Pacific Islander, American Indian or Alaska Native, Black and African American, and Asian (Office of Civil Rights, 1997).

Culture, Race, Ethnicity and Health Disparities

Culture, race, and ethnicity become factors impacting health disparities when persons, because of their identified ethnicity, cultural and physical characteristics differentiating them from other people, causes others to treat them wrongfully. However, culture and race should have no effect on one's health. Attributing risk factors or health indicators associated with race and culture can correlate with decreases or increases in lifespan longevity and incidence of disease. Hence, in addressing health disparities, it is imperative that culture and race be a part of the discussion and the plan to facilitate change.

CULTURE AND RACE: A CASE SCENARIO

A Community-Based Example of Addressing Health Disparities

African American children who reside in low-income communities and are diagnosed with asthma could benefit from the early intervention of nurse-led school-based teams with a focus on health promotion. School nurses can be instrumental in managing the health of African American children diagnosed with childhood asthma within the school setting. By collaborating with other disciplines within school systems, African American children and their families and community-based health care providers, school nurses can effectively advocate for the stabilization of asthma symptoms within low-income populations.

Literature Review

Asthma is an inflammatory process of the airway that affects the lung tissue. In the US, asthma is one of the leading chronic illnesses diagnosed in adolescents and children. Children and adolescents who have asthma can experience early-morning and night-time coughing, wheezing, shortness of breath, and chest tightness (CDC, 2017b; Patel & Wood, 2019). However, these symptoms can occur at any time during the day as well. Children and adolescents diagnosed with asthma tend to have a family history of this respiratory disease. Others may have no identifiable cause for the development of respiratory complications indicative of asthma. Allergies have been correlated with asthma triggers, such as burning wood, mold, outdoor air pollution, grass, dust mites, pollen, or exposure to tobacco smoke or cockroach dander (CDC, 2017; Hinkle & Cheever, 2018). According to the American Academy of Pediatrics, asthma causes disease and health burdens and affects approximately 7 million children (AAP, 2017). The CDC (2018) noted that, within the US, approximately 7% of White children have asthma, while 16% of Black children have been diagnosed.

Biomarkers are characteristics that are used to evaluate and measure pharmacologic, biologic, and pathogenic responses to a therapeutic intervention (Haldar & Pavord, 2007; Pin et al., 1992; Pizzichini et al., 1997). For example, Pizzichini et al. (1997; see also Uwaezuoke et al., 2018) examined the time course of symptoms after one, two, three, seven, and twenty-one days of treatment with prednisone in persons with severe asthma exacerbation. Additionally, airway inflammatory changes were observed in sputum samples. Saliva and blood from ten patients and forced expiratory volume were measured over the course of one second (FEV1). By evaluating the latter biomarkers, prednisone doses could be monitored and adjusted to meet the needs of the patients, as well as their individual treatment plan. At this time, there are no specific biomarkers that can identify predictive disease phenotypes for children. Although there are some biomarkers for severe asthma, this remains an area of ongoing research.

Patel and Teach (2019) noted that asthma is one of the leading causes of emergency department visits and is the most common respiratory disease occurring during childhood. Although there have been significant advances in the medical management of childhood asthma, the continuum of care for children affected with asthma is a problem. Patel and Teach (2019) recommend that asthma care must go beyond the patient and provider relationship office visit to facilitate effective disease management.

Environmental Contaminants

The WHO (2020) estimates that 3.8 million deaths annually are associated with exposure to smoke in households from fuel and dirty cook stoves, while 4.2 million deaths are related to outdoor ambient pollution, such as fumes emitted from industries, cars, and trucks. Worldwide, 91% of the population resides in areas where air quality is poor (WHO, 2020).

When exposed to environmental pollutants, children are more vulnerable to the development of asthma. Children's physical activity and physiological makeup cause them to be more susceptible to the effects of pollution than are adults. Areas of air pollution studied in the literature have included industrial (e.g., aluminum smelter emissions, oil refineries) and outdoor pollution (Rodriguez-Villamizar, 2018; Stieb & Liu, 2014; Brand et al., 2016). Low-income children are more likely to reside near industrial areas within the inner city.

Children with asthma attending older school buildings in low-income areas may be exposed to environmental contaminants, such as chalkboard dust, poorly maintained indoor air filters, extremes of indoor temperature regulation, and the absence of air conditioning in humid weather. Additional school exposures to allergens can include school bus exhaust fumes; cleaning supplies, such as bleach; dust and pollen; animals within the classroom, such as rabbits or hamsters; room deodorizers; perfume; the smell of markers used during arts and crafts; and freshly cut grass and pollen exposure during outdoor activities (NIH, 2012b; NIH, 2012c; NAEPP, 2020).

Asthma Diagnosis

Health care providers can assess children and adolescents for asthma when they present with recurrent symptoms of wheezing, cough, chest tightness, and difficulty breathing. Spirometry tests are included in the assessment to determine if the diagnosis of asthma is conclusive. A child or adolescent experiencing worsening symptomatology of asthma (an asthmatic attack) can become increasingly anxious and fearful, as they are unable to breathe and clear mucous from their airway and lungs. Spirometry tests assess breathing and lung function. During spirometry tests, the child or adolescent is asked to blow out forcefully through a mouthpiece, and exhaled volume and airflow is measured. Spirometry measurements can also be completed before and after the use of a short-acting bronchodilator to assess the child's or adolescent's response to the medication. A bronchial challenge can be done to assess airway hyperactivity if the spirometry measurements are normal but the child or adolescent is symptomatic (NIH, 2012a; NIH 2021a).

The fractional exhaled nitric oxide (FeNO) measurement test is a noninvasive procedure that uses quantitative data to measure the amount of fractional nitric oxide (NO) in a person's exhaled breath. The FeNO is a means to estimate airway inflammation. The current National Asthma Education and Prevention Program Coordinating Committee (NAEPPCC, 2020) Expert Panel Report 4 (EPR-4), recommends that, for children age five years or older for whom spirometry tests cannot be completed, the FeNO measurement should be performed in addition to physical examination and the gathering of historical data to rule out a diagnosis of asthma. FeNO measurement should not be used in isolation as a singular diagnostic approach or as a predictor of worsening asthma symptoms. However, the FeNO measurement can be beneficial in the management of asthma when used as a means of monitoring a child's asthmatic health progression. For children aged zero to four years who present clinically with recurrent episodes of wheezing, FeNO should not be used as a means to predict the development of asthma.

Asthma Severity and Control

The severity of asthma symptoms experienced by a child or adolescent is assessed by the health care provider in the determination of therapy and disease management. The goal of treatment is to control the symptoms of wheezing, difficulty breathing, cough, and chest tightness, thereby achieving targeted spirometry readings. Asthma control must be regularly assessed and maintained in the home, school, and healthcare settings to adjust therapies as needed (NIH, 2007; NAEPP, 2020).

According to Nagakumar and Thomas (2017), most children diagnosed with asthma are classified as having mild or moderate symptoms. These children's asthma symptoms are often managed with inhaled corticosteroids (ICSs) and bronchodilators. Although therapy-resistant asthma rarely occurs in children, 5% to 10% of children with asthma can have poorly managed asthma with therapy. Causes of poor asthma symptom control can include: gastroesophageal reflux, poor adherence to the treatment regimen, obesity, chronic rhinosinusitis, psychological factors, ongoing exposure to allergens, and suboptimal inhaler techniques. Hence, these children may miss days of school and excessively visit the doctor's office or emergency department, and their families can experience excessive stress in their households as caretakers focus on the stabilization of the child's asthma symptoms (Nagakumar & Thomas, 2017).

Interventions for the mitigation of allergens for children are conditionally based on the origin of the allergen trigger. For example, if there are no identified indoor allergens, the child should not be prescribed allergy medications. However, if a child has sensitivities, for example, to cockroaches, dust mites, or rodents, a multicomponent allergen mitigation is indicated. In this case, a caregiver would be instructed to purchase mattress and pillow covers that are impermeable to dust mites and, in the case of roach or rodent infestations, exterminators should be used to mitigate the problem (NAEPP, 2020).

Risk and impairment are domains of severity and control of asthma symptoms. A child or adolescent exhibiting risks associated with asthma may have a decline in the function of their lungs, adverse effects to medications, or exacerbations of symptoms. Impairments consist of limitations in the ability of the child to function in their daily lives, given the recent intensity and frequency of asthma symptoms (NIH, 2007; NAEPP, 2020; Global Initiative for Asthma [GINA], 2018).

Medications

For adults, children, and adolescents, ICSs are preferred for long-term therapy. ICSs in combination with long-acting beta2-agonists (LABAs) are equally preferred options for children age five years and older to decrease the frequency of asthma exacerbations. Omalizumab (Xolair), an anti-IgE monoclonal antibody, was originally marketed as a drug to treat patients with allergen sensitivities. Omalizumab was recommended by the National Institute for Health and Care Excellence (NICE) to treat persistent allergic asthma in people age six years and older (Nagakumar & Thomas, 2017; NICE, 2018).

For children between the ages of zero and four years who have recurrent wheezing related to respiratory tract infections only, a short course of treatment with an ICS is indicated once the respiratory infection has been diagnosed. Short-acting beta agonists (SABA), such as albuterol sulfate (American Academy of Allergy, Asthma & Immunology [AAAAI], 2021), can be used on an as-needed basis for quick relief therapy. Children over the age of four years diagnosed with mild to moderate persistent asthma and prescribed a daily ICS treatment should not have increases in dosing with brief episodes of worsening symptoms (i.e., decreased peak flow). While children four years and older with moderate to severe persistent asthma are recommended formoterol for relief therapy and daily control of asthma symptoms, they are prescribed a single inhaler. The two recommended treatments for the latter population are: ICS-LABA, same dose for daily control, and SABA for quick symptom relief, or ICS, higher-dose, for daily control of asthma symptoms and SABA for quick therapeutic relief. For children aged 12 years and older who are diagnosed with mild persistent asthma symptomatology, the use of daily ICS and as-needed SABA is recommended. In the event that quick relief is needed for worsening asthma symptoms, an ICS and SABA can be used together (NAEPP, 2020).

Long-acting muscarinic antagonists (LAMA) should not be added to an ICS routine in comparison to adding LABA to ICS in children aged 12 years and older who are diagnosed with uncontrolled persistent asthma. However, if LABA is not used for uncontrolled persistent asthma, LAMA can be added to ICS controller therapy rather than maintaining the same dosing of ICS. Currently, for children aged 12 years and older who are diagnosed with uncontrolled persistent asthma, the EPR-4 recommends conditionally adding LAMA to ICS-LABA, rather than maintaining the same dose of ICS-LABA (NAEPP, 2020).

For children aged five years and older who are diagnosed with mild to moderate asthma, conditional administration of immunotherapy administered subcutaneously can be used as an adjunct therapy, according to the EPR-4, for standard pharmacotherapy for children who have asthma that is controlled upon the initiation and build-up phases of maintenance therapy. For children diagnosed with persistent allergic asthma, the EPR-4 recommends that sublingual immunotherapy not be used in treatment. Youths aged 18 years and older who have been diagnosed with persistent asthma and who have a high value on potential benefits to their quality of life and a small reduction in asthma exacerbations, bronchial thermoplasty (BT) can be a treatment option. Additionally, for youths with a low value on harms with short-term asthma symptoms that have worsened with long-term side effects, BT can also be considered as a treatment (NAEPP, 2020).

When children and adolescents require treatment for asthma exacerbations, prehospital protocol includes: administration of oxygen and albuterol by emergency medical services (EMS). EMS personnel are permitted to administer oral systemic corticosteroids and anticholinergics with medical support and guidance (NIH, 2007; NAEPP, 2020). The NAEPP guidelines (NAEPP, 2020) recommend the addition of levalbuterol and heliox, or magnesium sulfate, if exacerbations do not respond to initial treatments. The use of oral corticosteroids is also recommended. Providers are advised to inform patients and their family members to not double the dose for at-home ICS, and that anticholinergics should be used during emergency care outside of the hospital only by EMS. Health care providers are to consider prescribing an ICS at the time of discharge (NIH, 2007; NAEPP, 2020).

Treatment

Treatment regimens for asthma tend to be devised by health care providers based on the global asthma severity category as intermittent or persistent (Everhart et al., 2018). The NAEPP developed guidelines for asthma that included changes to the following four areas: assessment monitoring, patient education, control of environmental factors and other conditions that can affect asthma, and medications (NIH, 2007, 2012, 2020). At times, children and adolescents will require modifications to their individual asthma management plans. The Stepwise Approach for the Management of Asthma applies current evidenced-based treatment to the care of children and adolescents diagnosed with asthma in varied age groups. Each step for the Stepwise Approach addresses the management of comorbidities, environmental controls, and patient education (i.e., self-management). Medication dosages will be adjusted, or *stepped up*, based on the symptoms the child or adolescent is exhibiting, or conversely *stepped down* (AAAAI, 2018).

Stepwise Approach for the Management of Asthma

The Stepwise Approach guidelines are asthma-control diagrams that are meant to assist health care providers and patients with asthma management, including making patient–provider decisions with the goal of stabilizing asthma symptoms. Health care providers escalate treatment interventions to a higher step or deescalate (lower step) treatment in asthma symptom management. The lower step is maintained once the child's or youth's asthma has been controlled for at least three consecutive months. According to the EPR-4, for children's and youth's asthma, diagnosed as persistent and requiring treatment at step two or above, health care providers will follow current treatment guidelines based on the patient's treatment-response history. For children and youths diagnosed with persistent asthma and using alternative treatments that have an inadequate response to asthma treatment, the EPR-4 recommends that the alternative treatment be discontinued and replaced with a preferred treatment at the same step level without stepping up to a higher level (NAEPP, 2020).

Financial Implications for Underinsured Low-Income Children

Fung et al. (2014) studied financial barriers experienced by 769 parents of children diagnosed with asthma. The children were aged 4 to 11 years old. Excluded from the study were children prescribed long-term corticosteroids or omalizumab. Fung et al. (2014) found that commercially insured parents with incomes at or less than 250% of the federal poverty level (FPL), in comparison with parents below 250% FPL receiving public subsidies, were more likely to delay bringing their children to the emergency department or health care provider's office. These parents were more likely to borrow money to cover the cost of health care cost-sharing (co-pays). Meanwhile, parents with incomes below the FPL were more likely to bring their children experiencing asthma-related complications to the emergency department or health care provider's office. These parents did not have health care cost-sharing because their insurance was covered by public subsidies. The delay in treatment was correlated with lower out-of-pocket costs.

Caregivers of Low-Income Children Diagnosed with Asthma

Everhart et al. (2018) conducted a study of 59 participants, all caregivers for children diagnosed with asthma. Of the 59 caregivers, 90% were African American/Black, had a child(ren) diagnosed with asthma, and resided within urban areas. The children were aged 7–12 years. The study results indicated that, when caregivers reported feeling unsafe in their neighborhood as a result of neighborhood violence, familial stress was heightened. Interestingly, caregivers reported that affected children's asthma symptoms increased in severity when the children faced conditions of heightened stress.

Nurses and School Systems

In 2016, H.R. 4662, the School-Based Asthma Management Program Act, was developed with the goal of improving school and health-related outcomes for children diagnosed with asthma (AAAAI, 2016). According to the CDC (2017a), in a classroom of approximately 30 children, three of those children are likely to have been diagnosed with asthma. The CDC (2017b) notes that "low-income populations, minorities and children living in inner cities experience more emergency department visits, hospitalizations, and deaths due to asthma than the general population."

In the US, lost school days associated with asthma total 10.5 million yearly, along with a total of $56 billion in health care costs (AAAAI, 2016). When asthma management education is provided by school nurses, these numbers can be reduced. Education, with emphasis on the recognition of early signs and symptoms of asthma and the use of an asthma plan, may help reduce the need for emergency department visits and hospitalizations for children (AAAAI, 2016).

METHODOLOGY

Exemplar Case: Adam

The methodology used to explore the role of the school nurse in the management of childhood asthma is an exemplar case study known as "Adam." The following case study is hypothetical; therefore, ethical approval is not indicated. The example is not based on an actual patient case. The purpose of this exemplar is to demonstrate the importance of the school nurse's role as a patient advocate and collaborator of care within the school setting. The Appraisal of Guidelines Research and Evaluation (AGREE) Reporting Checklist (Brouwers, Kerkvliet, & Spithoff, 2016) has been applied in the development of this exemplar case with the examination of the population health of low-income African American children and associated community, family, and school factors that can impact chronic disease management. The NAEPP EPR-4 (2020; CDC, 2017a) have been used to explain the four guidelines for state programs to ensure that comprehensive asthma care is provided to children with asthma.

Adam Miller is a 7-year-old African American male residing within a three-family home owned by his 67-year-old grandmother. Three generations of the family reside in the home: a grandmother, a great-grandmother, and Adam and his parents. The home is located within a low-income neighborhood in an urban area that is two blocks from a recycling plant and dump. Adam began exhibiting symptoms of asthma two years ago. The symptoms consisted of coughing at night and shortness of breath with exertion. No one in the household smoked, and his parents regularly mopped the wood floors present throughout the home.

Within the last two months, Adam missed 14 days of school related to emergency department visits and two hospitalizations, each with lengths of stay of three to four days. At school the nurse noticed that Adam was using his quick-relief inhaler, albuterol (Proventil), twice a week. Adam was requesting the inhaler shortly after arriving to school. Prior to recent hospitalizations, Adam used the quick-relief inhaler before outdoor recess only.

The school nurse called Adam's mother and requested she come by the school to meet with her to discuss Adam's worsening asthma symptoms. Adam's mother agreed to meet and arrived at the school within one hour. The school nurse provided an asthma information sheet to Adam's mother that contained online resources about medications, exposure to allergens, and environmental pollutants. The nurse also discussed with Adam's mother her recognition of changes in symptoms that could indicate that his asthma may be worsening, such as Adam gradually becoming short of breath as he played with his friends and disruption in sleep/rest patterns at home.

Adam's mother made an appointment for Adam to see his pediatrician while at the school nurse's office, and both she and the nurse discussed their concerns about Adam's asthma with the pediatrician in a shared telephone consultation at that time. Adam's mother shared, "Adam's asthma has always been well controlled. We keep the floors mopped; there are no throw rugs and no pets in our home. I can't understand it. Why is he having these symptoms?" The pediatrician concurred with Adam's mother's statements and requested that the school nurse call his office if Adam had any changes in his condition while at school. Adam was brought to the pediatrician's office for an appointment by his mother at the end of the meeting with the nurse.

Exemplar Case Progression: Two Weeks Later

During recess on the playground, Adam becomes short of breath. His teacher leaves the other children with the paraprofessional and immediately escorts Adam to the school nurse's office. Adam is provided his inhaler, and his symptoms subside. However, Adam continues to cough forcefully. Adam, upon inquiry by the nurse as to why he appears so sleepy, shares, "I have a hard time sleeping at night. Sometimes I breathe heavy." Adam's teacher shared with the nurse that Adam had missed two days of school this week.

The school nurse, concerned about the change in the severity of Adam's asthma symptoms and poor control, called Adam's pediatrician to inquire if consultation with an asthma specialist was being considered. The school nurse also called Adam's parents to inform them of the discussion with the pediatrician. During the phone call, Adam's parents shared that Adam had a visiting nurse (community health nurse), but services were discontinued after all family members received education on asthma management and could demonstrate understanding of the use of the medications, a Stepwise Approach Asthma Management Plan diagram was reviewed, and equipment was secured in the home (e.g., nebulizer, spacer). The school nurse requested written permission to talk with the community health nurse regarding the progression of Adam's asthma care while services were provided. Adam's frequent absences from school were discussed between the nurse and the school social worker.

During a conversation with the community health nurse regarding Adam's asthma management and eventual discharge from home care services, the school nurse was informed that Adam and his parents had received instruction on spacer- and inhaler-use techniques. Observed by the community health nurse several times, Adam and his parents were able to effectively demonstrate the appropriate techniques. Additionally, signs and symptoms of worsening asthma had been reviewed with the family, along with instructions on the use of a spirometer. The length of time for services provided by the home care agency was 30 days.

A meeting was convened seven days later with Adam's parents, the social worker, school nurse, teacher, school psychologist, and principal. The school nurse facilitated the meeting with a focus on asthma stabilization and the investigation of community supports and resources to help Adam and his parents. Adam's pediatrician was unavailable for participation in the meeting at that time, but had informed the school nurse that consultation with an asthma specialist had been initiated.

During the school meeting, Adam's teacher shared that, while he was engaged in classroom activities, he was frequently noted to be coughing upon arrival to school. The coughing typically subsided as the school day progressed. The school nurse concurred with the teacher's observations and shared Adam's recent increased meter-dosed inhaler (MDI) use during the school day with the team and Adam's parents. Adam's current use of an albuterol MDI with a chamber spacer prior to exertional activities was effective. However, given his recent need for additional dosing secondary to a verbal report of shortness of breath experienced early in the academic day, collaborative work was necessary to identify potential asthma triggers.

Adam's parents shared how they were concerned about their son's asthma exacerbations. Climatic changes (extremes of hot and cold temperatures) and pollen were reported by his parents to be primary triggers for Adam. His asthma had been otherwise stable since diagnosis at five years of age. The nurse shared upon consultation with Adam's pediatrician that a past medical history of well-managed asthma was confirmed and that the community health nurse verified that the family and Adam had been educated on the basics of asthma management.

The school nurse requested for Adam to be escorted from the classroom to join the meeting. Adam arrived to the meeting, and the school nurse explained that everyone was present to help find the cause of his worsening asthma. The nurse asked Adam if he could remember times during the day when he experienced coughing and difficulty breathing. Adam nervously responded, "I don't know why I have a hard time breathing. I am ok." The nurse thanked Adam for sharing. The meeting concluded with the plan to continue to monitor Adam in the school and home settings.

The School System's Role in Asthma Management

The NAEPP EPR-3 (2007; NAEPP, 2020; CDC, 2017a) identified four guidelines for state programs to ensure that comprehensive asthma care is provided to children with asthma. These guidelines were formulated to ensure that people with asthma, their caregivers, medical providers, and schools receive evidenced-based information on the management of this respiratory disease, thereby ensuring that children with asthma are assessed, correctly diagnosed, have environmental triggers identified, and have medications prescribed to stabilize their condition(s). The NAEPP EPR-4 guidelines (National, Heart, Lung, and Blood Institute, 2020a) began being developed in 2018 and were completed in 2020. These four guidelines represent an update to the NAEPP EPR-3 guidelines. The current goals of maintaining the health and well-being of children and adolescents diagnosed with asthma with evidenced-based treatment remain at the forefront. The four guidelines include:

1. Teach people with asthma how to manage their condition through "intensive asthma self-management education."
2. Ensure that people with asthma are connected to providers who can provide medical management that adheres to the NAEPP EPR-3 (and now NAEPP EPR-4, 2020) guidelines.

3. Teach caregivers, such as family members, school staff, and home visitors, about appropriate asthma management.
4. Provide information about evidence-based policies supportive of asthma control to people concerned about asthma, for example, informing them about the importance of good indoor air quality and the reduction of asthma triggers in places where people with asthma live, work, and play. (CDC, 2017a; CDC, 2017b)

Identifying Adam's Trigger(s)

The school nurse facilitated team collaboration among school and community-based providers by arranging meetings and conversations that addressed Adam's poorly controlled asthma. Academically and from a psychosocial perspective, the school, parents, and community-based providers, with the leadership provided by the school nurse, developed an action plan that addressed Adam's immediate health need of asthma stabilization and reduction of symptoms. Societally, when potential health equity issues are not addressed, worsening illness and disease will persist.

Five days after the meeting at the school, Adam presented to the school nurse's office after exiting the school bus in the morning. He was short of breath and wheezing and required the use of his albuterol inhaler. As Adam sat in the nurse's office, his symptoms resolving, he shared with the nurse that his great-grandmother, who had cancer, was dying at home. Adam began to cry and once again became short of breath. His breathing became increasingly more labored, and the nurse notified the school's secretary in the main office to call 911.

Adam's pediatrician was notified by the school nurse that he was being sent to the hospital for an increase in asthma symptom severity, after the unsuccessful intervention of the use of the bronchodilator albuterol. The nurse then notified Adam's parents by phone that their son would be sent to the hospital. While monitoring and assessing Adam's breathing, the nurse awaited the arrival of the ambulance. As Adam's breathing again stabilized, the nurse realized that the exacerbation of Adam's symptoms was likely related to stress that he was experiencing because his great-grandmother was ill.

Adam was transported to the hospital by ambulance, and after receiving albuterol nebulizer treatments, he stabilized. Adam's healthcare provider admitted him to the hospital for 48-hour observation to ensure his asthma exacerbation was well controlled. The school nurse asked Adam's parents' permission to visit them and their son at the hospital.

Upon arrival to the hospital, the school nurse informed Adam's parents of her observations of Adam's asthma symptoms worsening as he shared that his great-grandmother was dying. The parents confirmed that Adam's great-grandmother was receiving hospice services in the family home. Adam frequently slept with his great-grandmother and had continued to do so even as she became ill.

The school nurse provided support to Adam's parents. The nurse also explained how the stress of Adam's great-grandmother's illness may have contributed to the worsening of Adam's asthma symptoms. The parents shared this finding with Adam's pediatrician. After identifying Adam's trigger(s), a behavioral health consultation was made for the family, and a mental health provider met with Adam and his parents.

Additionally, the school nurse learned from Adam's parents that his school bus stop had been changed to a new site in the last six months. The new site was two blocks away from the family home in front of a recycling plant and dump. The debris from the landfill were also a potential trigger for Adam's asthma. The latter information was also provided to Adam's pediatrician.

Three days after Adam was discharged from the hospital, another school team meeting was arranged by the school nurse. Supportive services were put in place for Adam to have play therapy with the school psychologist. Adam transitioned to his parents' bed, and eventually to his own bedroom, as his great-grandmother received hospice care at home. The school nurse also facilitated the change of Adam's bus stop location with the bus company.

Considering Adam's frequent use of his albuterol inhaler, the recent hospitalizations, and the lack of control of his symptoms, Adam was started on a twice-daily regimen of a low-dose ICS, his inhaler technique was reviewed, and a follow-up visit was scheduled in two weeks to see how he was doing. With the support from the health care team and the use of his ICS, Adam's asthma gradually stabilized.

One month after the interventions were initiated, Adam's great-grandmother died. However, with the school-based supportive services in place, Adam had no further episodes of wheezing and shortness of breath in school and used his MDI for pre-medication only prior to recess while continuing with the low-dose ICS. The school nurse continued to collaborate with school staff, Adam's health care team, and his parents to assess and monitor the effectiveness of his asthma regimen.

School Nurses

School nurses are instrumental in ensuring that policies are in place within schools that protect and facilitate healthy environments for children with asthma and other health problems. The identification of children at risk for respiratory diseases like asthma begins with education of school staff about the disease and its impact on children and families. In May 2012, the Coordinated Federal Action Plan to Reduce Racial and Ethnic Asthma Disparities under the President's task force noted that

approximately 7 million children aged 0 to 17 in the US have asthma, with poor and minority children suffering a greater burden of the disease. Asthma persists into adulthood and the costs to society are high: medical expenses associated with asthma are estimated to be $50 billion annually. (NIH, 2012, p. 1)

The American Lung Association (2012) developed a model policy for school districts on stock bronchodilators that is followed in the 50 US states and the District of Columbia. With this model policy, students diagnosed with asthma can carry and use inhalers. Schools, with written healthcare provider orders, can have a stock of medications available in the event that students develop asthma symptoms.

School nurses, in collaboration with other professionals, can coordinate the academic, social-emotional, and health care needs of children. Working with children diagnosed with asthma, the school nurse must not only be knowledgeable of this respiratory disease process, but also understand how this chronic condition can affect children's lives. For Adam, the risk factors and environmental triggers for his asthma were not related to his racial-minority status or where he resided, but his emotional vulnerability as a child experiencing the dying process of a significant person in his life.

CONCLUSION

Nurses, by virtue of their professional training, are skilled in the assessment and management of respiratory conditions like asthma. Children with asthma experience chronic inflammation of the airway from this heterogeneous disease (GINA, 2015, 2018). They have excess mucous production, mucosal edema, and hyperresponsiveness leading to the clinical symptoms of dyspnea, cough, wheezing, and chest tightness (Hinkle & Cheever, 2018). Nurses working in school systems can assess and evaluate the management of children's asthma by asking parents and caregivers, in the presence of the child, the following questions:

1. How often is the quick-relief (emergency) inhaler used?
2. Does the child wake up early in the morning or late at night with difficulty breathing, chest tightness, wheezing, or coughing?
3. Has the child required unscheduled asthma care, such as emergency department visits or visits to the health care provider's office?
4. Has the child been having difficulty with asthma symptoms while running or playing at school or at home?
5. Do you or your child feel as if their asthma symptoms have worsened despite using medications?
6. Are there any stressful events the child may have witnessed or is experiencing at home?

By asking these questions, the school nurse can help families understand when and why symptoms of asthma are worsening and whether or not immediate intervention is needed. The nurse, in the role of educator to school staff, children (in the classroom), parents, and community-based providers can provide evidence-based information about asthma. There are also validated evidenced-based practice questionnaires that the school nurse can use to obtain information about a child's or adolescent's asthma condition, such as the Asthma Control Questionnaire, the Asthma Control Test, and the Asthma Therapy Assessment Questionnaire; these resources can help facilitate the development of asthma management and treatment plans (NHLBI, 2007). Through health promotion and collaborative work within school systems, children with asthma can be identified as being at risk for worsening asthma symptoms, and interventions can be implemented to assist these children and their families with asthma management. School nurses interested in pursuing nationally recognized certification for asthma can take an examination offered through the National Asthma Certification Board and become a designated Certified Asthma Educator (AE-C). School nurses can obtain more details about asthma certification at www.naecb.com.

Within the US, children's health can be affected by the zip code in which they reside, the school systems they attend, their immediate environment, socioeconomic status (SES), and their familial and community-based supports.

Although these factors can impact asthma stabilization, school nurses must examine other factors that can affect children with asthma, such as heightened stress. School systems can be instrumental in the identification of vulnerable populations and health equity issues. Nurses, social workers, health care providers, teachers, administrators, and community allies (i.e., community health nurses, landlords) can help improve health outcomes in children with asthma by implementing interventions that support and teach families how to navigate systems to bring about environmental change and stabilization of asthma symptomatology.

CASE STUDY DISCUSSION QUESTIONS

Directions: After reading the case study about Adam, read each question or statement below and discuss the case study progression and outcome.

1. Sometimes caregivers are unaware of how to manage and protect children and youths with asthma in the home environment from potential asthmatic triggers. In Adam's case, was this a concern with his parents?
2. School nurses are just one example of a profession that can be equipped with education about asthma management and current guidelines to ensure the health and safety of children and adolescents in school systems. What are other professions that also can help in the management and abatement of asthma for children and adolescents attending schools within the US?
3. What questions could have been asked of Adam to identify his worsening asthmatic symptoms earlier?
4. Adam slept with his great-grandmother prior to her becoming ill, rather than sleeping in his own room. Culturally, is this an occurrence that normally happens in families?
5. Is it important to examine familial, peer related, and academic stressors in the care of children and youths diagnosed with asthma?
6. How can school nurses and other professionals working with children and youths diagnosed with asthma who reside in low-income areas advocate for healthy living, neighborhood, and school environments?
7. Is it imperative that professionals working with children and adolescents diagnosed with asthma be aware of the guidelines proposed by the NAEPPCC EPR-4?

8. Communication with caregivers and health care providers is essential in advocating for children and youths diagnosed with asthma and attending schools in the US. Should asthma and other diseases impacting children's and youths' functionality be regularly discussed in interdisciplinary meetings? Should these meetings regularly include the child and adolescent?

CULTURE, RACE, AND HEALTH DISPARITIES

Culture and race have historically had an impact on health disparities within the US. Be it hypertension, teen pregnancy, sexually transmitted infections, or diabetes management, culture and race must be researched to identify potential health improvements. In the identification of gaps in treatment that impact race and culture, a resolution to the eradication of disease, illness, or syndrome can be explored and amended.

Culture and race data are often convoluted by what is reported by the nightly news, newspapers, and in social media. Hence, it is imperative that empirical data be obtained and current research findings validated to ensure that race and culture are not exploited to control a societal theme. For example, with teen pregnancy; as numbers of pregnant teens decreased in the US in 2016 and 2017, all races, not just ethnic minorities, were positively impacted (CDC, 2019a).

Breast Cancer, Teen Pregnancy, and Diabetes Health Promotion

Breast Cancer

During 2015–2017, women aged 50–70 years residing in the US (5.3%) had never been informed by a healthcare provider that they had the diagnosis of breast cancer. According to the National Center for Health Statistics (CDC, 2019b), Hispanic women compared to White women were 3.2% more likely to be informed that they had breast cancer, while White women were 6.1% more likely to be informed by a healthcare provider of a cancer diagnosis. Black women were 3.6% more likely to be informed of a breast cancer diagnosis. Hence, statistically, White women have been more likely to benefit from health promotion and the early diagnosis of breast cancer. Thus, White women were more likely than Hispanic and Black women to have positive breast cancer outcomes and survival rates.

Yedjou et al. (2019) noted that breast and skin cancers are the most common malignancies affecting women within the US. Black women, despite the innovations in screening, detection, and diagnosis are (Tammemagi, 2007; Hirschman et. al., 2007) more likely to not receive adequate treatment in comparison to White women. Asian women that have recently migrated to the US tend to have lower rates of breast cancer, than Asian women who have resided in the US for several years. However, the 5-year survival rate for Asian-American women is the same for White women. Hispanic women have a lower incidence of breast cancer than non-Hispanic white women (Howlader et al., 2014; Yedjou et al., 2019).

Teenage Pregnancy

Since 2009, there has been a gradual decline in teenagers giving birth within the US. In 2017, for females aged 15–19 years, the national birth rate was 18.8 births per 1,000 (194,377), a decrease of 7% (209,809) since 2016. This decrease was notably seen among the following racial and ethnic minority groups: American Indian, Alaskan, and Black teenagers (6%), Asian teenagers (15%), White teenagers (8%), Hispanic teenagers (9%), and Native Hawaiian or Pacific Islander teenagers (11%; CDC, 2019c). The latter data is evidence that teen pregnancy is not purely, an ethnic-minority issue, but impacts all families in the US. Teenage mothers statistically, are more likely to smoke during pregnancy, resulting in low- birthweight infants, and less likely to receive prenatal care.

Diabetes

Data gathered from the National Health Interview Survey administered January through June of 2018 noted that Hispanics (12.4%) were more likely to be diagnosed with diabetes, while Blacks were 11.5% and Whites were 7.7%. In the US, an estimated 34.2 million people, or 10.5% of the population, have diabetes, with 26.9 million (26.8 million adults) being formally diagnosed. An estimated 7.3 million people are believed to be undiagnosed (CDC, 2020a). Given the data that have been tabulated nationally in the US on the prevalence of diabetes and its impact on racial- and ethnic-minority communities, education is needed to improve knowledge of prevention. Current numbers are evidence of a health crisis complicated by poor diet, lack of exercise, obesity, and other factors that impact the likelihood that this health disparity will persist if this crisis is not addressed at a state and national level.

Hypertension

By the age of 55, approximately three-fourths of African Americans are likely to have developed hypertension compared to 40% of White women and 55% of White men (American Heart Association [AHA], 2020). Research examining factors that contribute to hypertension among African Americans have identified stress as a link. African Americans are more likely to reside in impoverished neighborhoods, to have experienced childhood trauma associated with living in high-crime areas, and to encountered discrimination (AHA, 2020). The last aspect coincides with cardiovascular risk factors, such as obesity, tobacco use, diabetes mellitus, sleep disorders (i.e., obstructive sleep apnea), and poor intake of nutritional foods (i.e., fresh fruits and vegetables, nuts, and other plant-based foods) related to living in neighborhoods with poor access to quality food sources.

In 2017, the AHA, with the endorsement of the American College of Cardiology, developed a scientific statement on cardiovascular health in African Americans. Recognizing that African Americans have not been equally impacted by the reductions nationally in cardiovascular mortality and incidence, the AHA examined causes of this societal problem. For the purpose of their research, African Americans were explored as one of the oldest nonnative racial groups residing in the US. Unlike ethnic minorities with African ancestry, such as persons originating from Latin America and the Caribbean, African Americans originally were brought to this country by means of the transatlantic slave trade (AHA, 2020); their migration was involuntary. Since that time, African Americans have endured discrimination and social injustices.

Race-specific guidelines for treatment of hypertension among African Americans are warranted because current use of angiotensin-converting enzyme inhibitors (ACE inhibitors) to treat this population are not as effective as using diuretics and beta blockers. Even using ACE inhibitors in combination with beta blockers have been ineffective (AHA, 2017). Yet, these are the medications that continue to be prescribed to persons of African descent. Hence, the healthcare community, by adhering to guidelines that have been proven scientifically to not always be effective for African Americans, contributes to poor hypertension outcomes, such as organ failure. While African Americans must themselves become knowledgeable of their own health care and disease management through interventions, such as weight loss, dietary changes, exercise, drug use, smoking cessation, and decrease or absence of alcohol intake, like most Americans, they too are reliant on the expertise of health care professionals to help them make informed, educated lifestyle changes.

The Joint National Committee on Prevention, Detection, Evaluation, and Treatment of High Blood Pressure's eighth report (James et al., 2014) has provided recommendations for blood pressure management for African Americans. One of those recommendations was to use a thiazide-type diuretic and calcium channel blocker as the initial treatment for hypertension for members of this community. There was even discussion on increasing the systolic blood pressure threshold specifically for African Americans to 150 mm Hg if they are greater or less than 60 years of age. Of concern is that these suggested treatment regimens, particularly the high systolic blood pressure, can lead to the development of organ failure (James et al., 2014; Wright et al., 2014). Currently, lower national blood pressure guidelines (i.e., a normal blood pressure is less than 120/80 mm Hg) set forth in November 2017 by the American College of Cardiology are being followed and prevent organ failure (ACC, 2017).

Sickle Cell Anemia

Sickle cell anemia is a disease manifested by the abnormal shape of erythrocytes (red blood cells). Red blood cells are normally round in shape. In sickle cell anemia, the red blood cells are shaped like crescent moons (or sickles) and, as a result of their shape, get stuck together and impair normal blood flow (Hinkle & Cheever, 2018). The anemia becomes problematic because of the reduction in mature red blood cells in circulation because the crescent-moon-shaped cells break apart and die easily as a result of their structure. With a reduction in red blood cells in the body, oxygenation is impacted, and affected persons become fatigued. Pain is experienced because of the impairment in blood flow.

Persons affected with sickle cell anemia can have multiple complications that can include: delayed puberty and growth, infections, joint and bone damage, stroke, vision problems (blindness), gall stones, complications in pregnancy (e.g., clots, miscarriage, low birth weight, and hypertension), inflammation of the feet and hands, acute chest syndrome, pulmonary hypertension, organ damage, leg ulcerations, and priapism. Acute exacerbations are painful, and affected persons may require treatment interventions, such as blood transfusions, blood thinners (e.g., prophylactic heparin to prevent deep vein thrombosis), intravenous fluids, dietary modifications, and pain medication. Sickle cell disease is genetic and involves a mutation (HbS) in hemoglobin. In the US, sickle cell anemia primarily impacts Black people (NIH, 2020b; Shah & Dwivedi, 2020).

The sickle cell anemia gene, HbS, is inherited in persons of African descent, but can also be present in people from Aboriginal tribes in India and people from the Middle East and the Mediterranean. Current treatment for sickle cell anemia includes transfusion therapy (red blood cell transfusions), pharmacologic therapy (i.e., hydroxyurea), hematopoietic stem cell transplant (requires a compatible donor), and supportive therapy (i.e., nonsteroidal anti-inflammatory drugs, opioids, hydration, rest, folic acid, blood thinners, and activity as tolerated to prevent deep vein thrombosis). At this time, the only known cure for sickle cell disease is the transplantation of bone marrow and blood transfusion, and very few people have had this procedure as it requires a compatible donor (there is a low number of racial- and ethnic-minority donors) and insurance access to pay for the procedure and aftercare (Hinkle & Cheever, 2018; National Heart, Lung, and Blood Institute, 2020).

Racial and Ethnic Minorities and Organ and Bone Marrow Transplantation

At this time, African Americans are the largest group of racial minorities on waiting lists awaiting organ transplants. In 2019, White Americans consisted of 47.6% of recipients of transplants, while African Americans made up 25.8%. African Americans currently compose 12.7% of the US population (DHHS, Office of Minority Health, 2020). The number of White Americans on organ transplant lists is approximately 1.4 times greater than that of Blacks. Furthermore, African Americans in 2019 made up 12.5% of organ donors, however, 74.5% of donor organs in 2019 were from deceased Black organ donors (DHHS, Office of Minority Health, 2020). The latter is indicative of a health disparity given that the majority of donor organs came from Black people, however, Blacks themselves, are less likely to receive these organs.

In 2019, 6,755 (21.0%) Black Americans were recipients of transplants in the US, as were 21,248 (54.5%) White Americans (US DHHS, 2020). Currently,

African Americans tend to have higher rates of diabetes and hypertension, both of which increase the risk of organ failure. It is therefore imperative that health promotion strategies be focused on the prevention of hypertension and diabetes in this population in order to effectively address the health disparities associated with organ transplantation. Additionally, Blacks must be provided education on the value of organ donation in sustaining all lives and that organ donation can occur while one is alive and not just in death. Advocacy is also indicated for fair access of African Americans to donor organs.

Health Disparities among American Indians and Alaska Natives

Jacobs-Wingo et al. (2016) tracked the leading causes of death among American Indian and Alaska Native populations that resided in urban areas in the US. Data were gathered during 1999–2009 and focused on the comparison of causes of death among White Americans who resided in urban areas with those of American Indians and Alaska Natives in both urban and rural locations. To avoid racial misclassification in the death certificates, Indian Health Service patient registration records were linked with the National Death Index.

Upon exploring the data, the five leading causes of death for American Indian and Alaska Native populations were heart disease, cancer, unintentional injury, diabetes, and chronic liver disease and cirrhosis. In comparison to White Americans living in urban areas, the American Indian and Alaska Native populations had higher rates of death in all five of the identified conditions. The rates of death were similar even when American Indian and Alaska Native populations resided in rural areas. Further research is needed to understand clinical interventions and public health initiatives that can be practiced to help reduce these health disparities and examine contributing conditions and behaviors (Jacobs-Wingo et al., 2016).

American Indians and Alaska Natives: Women and Sexual Health

Higher rates of sexually transmitted infections exist among racial and ethnic minorities in comparison to White Americans. Unemployment, no insurance or being underinsured, and low education levels are contributing factors to racial and ethnic minorities not receiving adequate sexual health care. Currently, sexually transmitted infections are a health equity issue within the US (CDC, 2020b).

Cahn et al. (2019) examined data from the National Survey of Family Growth for women aged 15–44 years who self-identified as Alaska Native or American Indian (n = 819, 78% of participants), or as non-Hispanic White women (n = 6,196). Sexual health services data were collected from 2006 to 2010. The data indicated higher rates in the following areas for Alaska Native and American Indian women in comparison to non-Hispanic White women: unplanned pregnancy and abortion were 1.5–2 times higher (Urban Indian Health Institute and Seattle Indian Health Board, 2010), sexually transmitted infections and human immunodeficiency virus (HIV) were 3–4 times higher (CDC, 2016a; 2016b), and teen birth rate was 1.6 times higher (Martin et al., 2017).

American Indian and Alaska Native women that reside in rural areas tend to live near Indian Health Services (IHS) and are more likely to have a health care provider that they had an appointment scheduled with during the past year. Meanwhile, women who lived in urban areas and did not have access to IHS tended to have more health disparities (Cahn et al., 2019; Moss, 2010; CDC, 2015). American Indian and Alaska Native women residing in urban areas within the US may benefit from the availability of culturally sensitive sexual health care in the reduction of health disparities.

Asian Americans: Discrimination and Health Disparities

A national probability-based phone survey was conducted from January 26 to April 9, 2017, by an independent firm. The survey was designed by the Robert Wood Johnson Foundation, National Public Radio, and the Harvard T.H. Chan School of Public Health. Within the original sample size of 3,453, Native Americans, Latinx, LGBTQ (lesbian, gay, bisexual, transgender, and queer/questioning), Asian Americans, African Americans, and White Americans were included. Data from 902 non-Hispanic White Americans and 500 Asian non-Hispanic Americans were reviewed as subsamples. The findings indicated that, while Asian Americans experienced discrimination in many aspects of their lives, prominent areas noted during the study were while seeking housing and with physical and mental health care. Of concern is that the discrimination experienced by Asian Americans in health care contributed to health disparities because affected persons were less likely to use health services (McMurtry et al., 2019).

Weng and Wolfe (2016) noted that, because historical trends have identified Asian Americans as a model minority group, there is minimal data addressing their health inequities. Lee et al. (2010) described the label **model minority** as the perception that Asian Americans have successfully adapted to American life because of their achievement of higher education and income levels in comparison to other minority groups. However, culture and linguistic differences among Asian Americans are factors that contribute to maltreatment and discrimination in healthcare (and other institutions). Weng et al. (2016), applying a sociocultural framework for health disparities, suggested that, when studying health disparities within the Asian American population, multiple factors can be encountered. Hence, it is imperative that data reference the macro, meso, and microsystem levels.

SUMMARY

Historically, the origins of one's culture and race can have implications for how they respond or do not respond to traditional medical approaches. Factors such as socioeconomics, trauma, stress, diet, discrimination, obesity, and environmental pollutants can all impact how people survive and thrive with regard to their health. Likewise, deterioration of health can occur when these factors are not eliminated or drastically reduced. The purpose of bringing recognition to health disparities and inequities is to encourage honest discussions of how we can call to account persons, laws, regulations, and organizations that affect vulnerable populations by impacting their health outcomes. It is also important to provide affected populations with preventive health care knowledge and access to evidenced-based healthcare and community resources to improve their own health outcomes.

THIS ALL SEEMS SO UNFAIR

Directions: Read each question and statement. Consider the words *fair* and *unfair*. Fairness, or being *fair*, refers to that which is just and without partiality. Meanwhile, *unfair* is not being founded upon what has been deemed just or equal.

1. The word "unfair" is rhetorical and based on access. Consider why health disparities exist, using the word "unfair" in your statement.
2. Given the unpredictability of life, it can be said that one's social status or lot in society is of their own choosing. Do you agree or disagree with this statement? Please explain.
3. Can organizations that promote science have discriminatory motives? Or, can they just be misinformed?
4. Why is it important for health care providers and professionals within communities to work together to enhance the mental and physical health of community members?
5. Do the circumstances under which a racial or ethnic minority group arrived to a country matter? How does this impact their experience with health inequities?
6. Can being treated differently from others impact one's health?
7. How can persons living in rural or impoverished communities be empowered to improve their personal health and the care they receive from healthcare systems (agencies or facilities) located in their neighborhoods?
8. Should health care professional organizations be held accountable for promoting bad science that can potentially harm minorities and socioeconomically deprived persons?
9. Is more diversity among health care professionals needed to improve and address health disparities and inequities?
10. Explain the differences between culture and race. How do these differences impact the ways that health care is delivered to all people?
11. Is treating persons differently because of their race or cultural background fair or unfair? Explain your response.

CASE STUDY: MODEL MINORITY

I have been an American citizen for ten years. I have a beautiful suburban home and a great job as a chemist for a prominent drug company. I still have an accent, but I have been told that I speak clearly, although it takes time to get used to how my voice sounds. I'm from Japan, and my accent is proudly attributed to my country of origin. Sometimes I do not feel accepted for who I am, but then more is expected of me. After all, I am educated, and I have straight hair and light skin. I fit in to some degree, but not really. But I know I am viewed as a model minority.

Discussion: Have persons who are identified as model minorities fully assimilated?

Figure 1. Sometimes the visions of the living get lost on the banks of the water

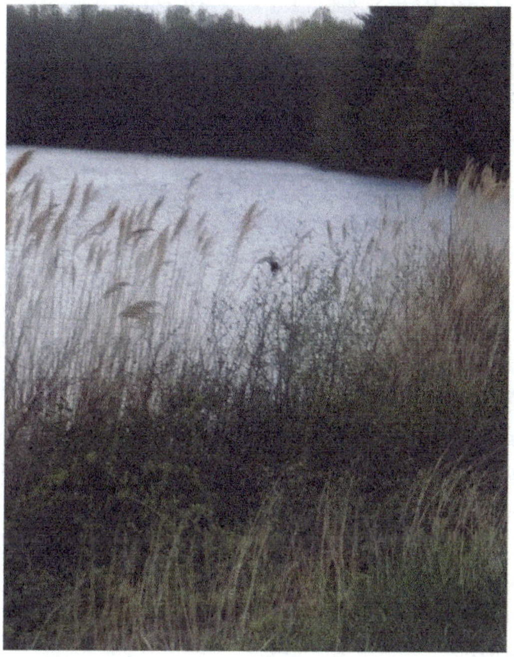

REFERENCES

Akinbami, L. J., Simon, A. E., & Rossen, L. M. (2016). Changing trends in asthma prevalence among children. *Pediatrics*, *137*(1), 107. doi:10.1542/peds.2015-2354 PMID:26451718

American Academy of Allergy, Asthma & Immunology. (2016). *School Asthma Management Plan Act*. https://www.aaaai.org/about-aaaai/advocacy/school-asthma-plan-act

American Academy of Allergy, Asthma & Immunology. (2018). *Follow the stepwise approach for asthma control*. https://www.aaaai.org/conditions-and-treatments/library/asthma-library/follow-stepwise-approach-for-asthma-control

American Academy of Allergy, Asthma & Immunology. (2020). *AAAAI allergy & medication guide*. https://www.aaaai.org/conditions-and-treatments/drug-guide/saba

American Academy of Pediatrics. (2017). Clinical tools to assess asthma control in children. *Pediatrics, 139*(1), 1–9. https://pediatrics.aappublications.org/content/139/1/e20163438

American College of Cardiology. (2017, November 13). *New ACC/AHA high blood pressure guidelines lower definition of hypertension*. https://www.acc.org/latest-in-cardiology/articles/2017/11/08/11/47/mon-5pm-bp-guideline-aha-2017

American Heart Association. (2017). *Cardiovascular health in African Americans: A scientific statement from the American Heart Association*. https://www.ahajournals.org/doi/pdf/10.1161/CIR0000000000000534

American Heart Association. (2020). *Is reducing stress the key to lowering heart disease among African Americans?* https://www.heart.org/en/news/2020/04/10/is-reducing-stress-the-key-to-lowering-heart-disease-among-AfricanAmericans

American Lung Association. (2012). *Model policy for school districts: Stock bronchodilators*. https://www.lung.org/assets/documents/asthma/model-policy-for-school.pdf

Brand, A., McLean, K. E., Henderson, S. B., Fournier, M., Liu, L., Kosatsky, T., & Smargiassi, A. (2016). Respiratory hospital admissions in young children living near metal Smelters, pulp mills and oil refineries in two Canadian provinces. *Environment International*, *94*, 24–32. https://www.doi.org/10.1016/j.envint.2016.052

Brouwers, M. C., Kerkvliet, K., & Spithoff, K. (2016). The AGREE Report Checklist: A tool to improve reporting of clinical guidelines. *British Medical Journal*, *352*, ill52. https://doi.org/10.1136/bmj.i1152

Cahn, M. A., Harvey, S. M., & Gonzales, K. (2019). Use of sexual health services among American Indian and Alaska Native women. *Women & Health*, *59*(9), 953–966. https://doi.org/10.1080/03630242.2019.1584144

Centers for Disease Control and Prevention. (2015). *2015 Indian Health Surveillance Report: Sexually Transmitted Diseases*. https://www.cdc.gov/std/statistics/ihs/18IHS-DEDP102_REPORT_STD_M_508.pdf

Centers for Disease Control and Prevention. (2016a). *HIV surveillance report.* https://www.cdc.gov/hiv/pdf/library/reports/surveillance/cdc-hiv-surveillance-report-2016-vol-28.pdf

Centers for Disease Control and Prevention. (2016b). *Sexually transmitted disease surveillance 2015.* U.S. Department of Health and Human Services. https://www.cdc.gov/std/stats16/CDC_2016_STDS_Report-for508WebSep21_2017_1644.pdf

Centers for Disease Control and Prevention. (2017a). *Strategies for addressing asthma in schools.* https://www.cdc.gov/asthma/pdfs/strategies_for_addressing_asthma_in_schools_508.pdf

Centers for Disease Control and Prevention. (2017b). *Learn how to control asthma.* https://www.cdc.gov/asthma/faqs.htm

Centers for Disease Control and Prevention. (2018). *Asthma in children.* https://www.cdc.gov/vitalsigns/childhood-asthma/

Centers for Disease Control and Prevention. (2019). *National Center for Health Statistics on Racial and Ethnic Disparities.* https://www.cdc.gov/nchs/data/factsheets/factsheet_disparities.htm

Centers for Disease Control and Prevention. (2020a). *National diabetes statistics report 2020: Estimates of diabetes and its burden in the United States.* https://www.cdc.gov/diabetes/pdfs/data/statistics/national-diabetes-statistics-report.pdf

Centers for Disease Control and Prevention. (2020b). *Sexually transmitted diseases (STDs)-STD health equity.* https://www.cdc.gov/std/health-disparities/default.htm

Everhart, R. S., Borschuk, A. P., Miadich, S. A., Barsell, J., & Heron, K. E. (2018). Caregiver daily experiences associated with child asthma symptoms. *American Journal of Health Behavior, 42*(2), 50–60. https://doi.org/10.5993/AJHB.42.2.5

Fung, V., Graetz, I., Galbraith, A., Hamity, C., Huang, J., Vollmer, W. M., Hsu, J., & Wu, A. C. (2014). Financial barriers to care among low-income children with asthma: Health care reform implications. *JAMA Pediatrics, 168*(7), 649–656. https://doi.org/10.1001/jamapediatrics.2014.79

Global Initiative for Asthma. (2015). *New global asthma strategy launched.* https://ginasthma.org/new-global-asthma-strategy-launched/

Global Initiative for Asthma. (2018). *2018 GINA report, global strategy for asthma management and prevention*. https://ginasthma.org/2018-gina-report-global-strategy-for-asthma-management-and-prevention

Haldar, P., & Pavord, I. D. (2007). Noneosinophilic asthma: A distinct clinical and pathologic phenotype. *Journal of Allergy & Clinical Immunology, 119*(5), 1043–1054. doi:10.1016/j.jaci.2007.02.042

Hinkle, J. L., & Cheever, K. H. (2018). *Brunner & Suddarth textbook of medical-surgical nursing* (14th ed.). Wolters Kluwer.

Hirschman, J., Whitman, S., & Ansell, D. (2007). The black:white disparity in breast cancer mortality: The example of Chicago. *Cancer Causes & Control, 18*(3), 323–333. doi:10.100710552-006-0102-y

Howlander, N., Noone, A. M., Krapcho, M., Garshell, J., Miller, D., Altekruse, S. F., Kosary, C. I., Yu, M., Ruhl, J., Tatalovich, Z., Mariotto, A., Lewis, D. R., Chen, H. S., Feuer, E. J., & Cronin, K. A. (2014). *Seer cancer statistics review 1975-2012*. National Cancer Institute. https://seer.cancer.gov/archive/csr/1975_2012/

Jacobs-Wingo, J. L., Espey, D. K., Groom, A. V., Phillips, L. E., Haverkamp, D. S., & Stanley, S. L. (2016). Causes and disparities in death rates among urban American Indian and Alaska Native populations, 1999–2009. *American Journal of Public Health, 106*, 906–914. https://doi.org/10.2105/AJPH.2015.303033

James, P. A., Oparil, S., Carter, B. L., Cushman, W. C., Dennison-Himmelfarb, C., Handler, J., Lackland, D. T., LeFevre, M. L., MacKenzie, T. D., Ogedegbe, O., Smith, S. C. Jr, Svetkey, L. P., Taler, S. J., Townsend, R. R., Wright, J. T. Jr, Narva, A. S., & Ortiz, E. (2014). Evidence-based guideline for the management of high blood pressure in adults: Report from the panel members appointed to the Eighth Joint National Committee (JNC 8). *Journal of the American Medical Association, 311*, 507–520. https://doi.org/10.1001/jama.2013.284427

Kim, J. S. (2015). Financial barriers to care among low-income children with asthma: Health care reform implications. *Pediatrics, 136*, S267. doi:10.1542/peds

Lee, S., Martinez, G., Ma, G. X., Hsu, C. E., Robinson, E. S., Bawa, J., & Juon, H.-S. (2010). Barriers to health care access in 13 Asian American communities. *American Journal of Health Behavior*, *34*(1), 21–30. https://doi.org/10.5993/AJHB.34.1.3

Martin, J. A., Hamilton, B. E., Osterman, M. J. K., Driscoll, A. K., & Mathews, T. J. (2017). Births: Final data for 2015. In National vital statistics reports, (p. 5). National Center for Health Statistics.

McMurtry, C. L., Findling, M. G., Casey, L. S., Blendon, R. J., Benson, J. M., Sayde, J. M., & Miller, C. (2019). Discrimination in the United States: Experiences of Asian Americans. *Health Services Research*, *54*, 1419–1430. https://dx.doi.org/10.1111/1475-6773.13225

Moss, M. P. (2010). American Indian health disparities: By the sufferance of Congress? *Hamline Journal of Public Law & Policy*, *32*(1), 58–81.

National Association of Social Work. (2012). *NASW standards for school social work services*. http://c.ymcdn.com/sites/www.sswaa.org/resource/resmgr/imported/naswschoolsocialworkstandards.pdf

National Asthma Education and Prevention Program. (2007). *Expert Panel Report 3, guidelines for the diagnosis and management of asthma*. https://www.nhlbi.nih.gov/files/docs/guidelines/asthsumm.pdf

National Asthma Educator Certification Board. (2018). *Certified asthma educator*. https://www.naecb.com/

National Heart, Lung, and Blood Institute. (2007). *National Asthma Education and Prevention Program- Export Panel Report 3: Guidelines for the diagnosis and management of asthma*. https://www.nhlbi.nih.gov/files/docs/guidelines/asthgdln.pdf

National Heart, Lung, and Blood Institute. (2020a). *Expert Panel Report 4 (EPR-4) Working Group: National Asthma Education and Prevention Program*. https://www.nhlbi.nih.gov/about/advisory-and-peer-review-committees/national-asthma-education-and-prevention-program-coordinating/EPR4-working-group

National Heart, Lung, and Blood Institute. (2020b). *Sickle cell disease*. https://www.nhlbi.nih.gov/health-topics/sickle-cell-disease

National Institute for Health and Care Excellence. (2018). *Omalizumab for treating severe persistent allergic asthma*. https://www.nice.org.uk/guidance/ta278

National Institutes of Health. (2007). *National asthma guidelines updated: New approaches for monitoring asthma control, expanded recommendations for children*. https://www.nih.gov/news-events/news-releases/national-asthma-guidelines-updated

National Institutes of Health. (2012a). *Asthma care quick reference: Diagnosing and managing asthma*. https://www.nhlbi.nih.gov/files/docs/guidelines/asthma_qrg.pdf

National Institutes of Health. (2012b). *Asthma disparities*. https://ptfceh.niehs.nih.gov/activities/asthma/index.htm

National Institutes of Health. (2012c). *President's Task Force on Environmental Health Risks to Children: Coordinated federal action plan to reduce racial and ethnic asthma disparities*. https://ptfceh.niehs.nih.gov/activities/assets/files/coordinated_federal_action_plan_to_reduce_racial_and_ethnic_asthma_disparities_508.pdf

National Institutes of Health. (2021a). *Asthma management guidelines: Focused updates 2020*. https://www.nhlbi.nih.gov/health-topics/asthma-management-guidelines-2020-updates

National Institutes of Health. (2021b). *Cultural respect*. https://www.nih.gov/institutes-nih/nih-office-director/office-communications-public-liaison/clear-communication/cultural-respect#:~:text=Culture%20is%20often%20described%20as,%2C%20geographic%2C%20or%20social%20groups

Patel, S. J., & Teach, S. J. (2019). Asthma. *American Academy of Pediatrics, 40*(11), 549–567. doi:10.1542/pir.2018-0282

Pin, I., Freitag, A. P., O'Byrne, P. M., Girgis-Gabardo, A., Watson, R. M., Dolovich, J., Denburg, J. A., & Hargreave, F. E. (1992). Changes in the cellular profile of induced sputum after allergen-induced asthmatic responses. *American Review of Respiratory Disease, 145*(6), 1265–1269. doi:10.1164/ajrccm/145.6.1265

Pizzichini, M. M., Pizzichini, E., Clelland, L., Efthimiadis, A., Mahony, J., Dolovich, J., & Hargreave, F. E. (1997). Sputum in severe exacerbations of asthma: Kinetics of inflammatory indices after prednisone treatment. *American Journal of Respiratory and Critical Care Medicine, 155*(5), 1501–1508. doi:10.1164/ajrccm.155.5.9154849

Rodríguez-Villamizar, L. A., Rojas-Roa, N. Y., Blanco-Becerra, L. C., Herrera-Galindo, V. M., & Fernández-Niño, J. A. (2018). Short-Term Effects of Air Pollution on Respiratory and Circulatory Morbidity in Colombia 2011-2014: A Multi-City, Time-Series Analysis. *International Journal of Environmental Research and Public Health, 15*(8), 1610. doi:10.3390/ijerph15081610

Shah, F., & Dwivedi, M. (2020). Pathophysiology and recent therapeutic insights of sickle cell disease. *Annals of Hematology, 99*, 925–935 https://doi-org.idm.oclc.org/10.1007/s00277-020-03977-9

Stieb, D., & Liu, L. (2014). Air quality impacts on health. In E. Taylor & A. McMillan (Eds.), Air quality management (pp. 141–166). Springer Publishing. https://doi.org/10.1007/978-94-007-7557-2_7.

Tammemagi, C. M. (2007). Racial-ethnic disparities in breast and gynecologic cancer treatment and outcomes. *Current Opinion in Obstetrics & Gynecology, 19*(1), 31–36. doi:10.1097/GCO.0b013e3280117cf8

Taylor, C., Lynn, P., & Bartlett, J. L. (2019). *Fundamentals of nursing: The art and science of person-centered care* (9th ed.). Wolters Kluwer.

United States Department of Health and Human Services. (2020). *Organ Procurement and Transplantation Network: National data*. https://optn.transplant.hrsa.gov/data/view-data-reports/national-data/

United States Department of Health and Human Services, Office of Minority Health. (2020). *Organ donation and African Americans*. https://minorityhealth.hhs.gov/omh/browse.aspx?lvl=4&lvlid=27

United States Department of the Interior. (1997). *Office of Civil Rights: Standards for maintaining, collecting, and presenting federal data on race and ethnicity*. https://www.doi.gov/pmb/eeo/directives/race-data#:~:text=The%20standards%20have%20five%20categories,%22Not%20Hispanic%20or%20Latino.%22

Urban Indian Health Institute. (2015). *About urban Indian health organizations*. http://www.uihi.org/about-urban-indian-health-organizations

Uwaezuoke, S., Ayuk, A., & Eze, J. (2018). Severe bronchial asthma in children: A review of novel biomarkers used as predictors of the disease. *Journal of Asthma and Allergy*, *11*, 11–18. https://doi.org/10.2147/JAA.S149577

Weng, S. S., & Wolfe, W. T. III. (2016). Asian American health inequities: An exploration of cultural and language incongruity and discrimination in accessing and utilizing the healthcare system. *International Public Health Journal*, *8*(2), 155–167.

World Health Organization. (2020). *Air pollution*. http://www9.who.int/airpollution/en/

Wright, J. T. Jr, Fine, L. J., Lackland, D. T., Ogedegbe, G., & Dennison Himmelfarb, C. R. (2014). Evidence supporting a systolic blood pressure goal of less than 150 mm Hg in patients aged 60 years or older: The minority view. *Annals of Internal Medicine*, *160*, 499–503. https://doi.org/10.7326/M13-2981

Yedjou, C. G., Sims, J. N., Miele, L., Noubissi, F., Lowe, L., Fonseca, D. D., Alo, R. A., Payton, M., & Tchounwou, P. B. (2019). Health and Racial Disparity in Breast Cancer. *Advances in Experimental Medicine and Biology*, *1152*, 31–49. https://doi.org/10.1007/978-3-030-20301-6_3

Chapter 4
Psychological Implications of Health Disparities

ABSTRACT

The psychological implications of health disparities are damaging as humans of different religions, genders, races, cultures, and socioeconomic backgrounds seek entry into healthcare systems and receive poor quality of treatment related to health care workers' and healthcare providers' conscious and unconscious biases. Linguistics, a cultural aspect of diversity, also impacts healthcare disparities, as language barriers affect health literacy. Psychologically impaired by both perceived and overt expressions of discrimination, affected persons can develop discomfort in seeking health care treatment secondary to a history of maltreatment by healthcare workers and providers. However, this pattern of maltreatment can be altered when healthcare workers are educated about unconscious biases and how, if not brought to awareness and removed from the daily interactions with others, they impact the physical and mental health of generations of people.

LEARNING OBJECTIVES

1. Discuss the allostatic load and its impact on low-income postpartum women.
2. Discuss how language barriers can impact health care delivery when not addressed.

DOI: 10.4018/978-1-7998-3874-6.ch004

3. Determine the psychological impact of racial, cultural, and religious discrimination to persons impacted.
4. Explain how low-income immigrant children are at risk for health disparities.
5. Explain why the lesbian, gay, bisexual, and transgender communities are impacted by societal discrimination.
6. Discuss the importance of having American Sign Language-certified interpreters in healthcare facilities.
7. Explain how discrimination can be a factor in a person's suicidal ideation.

Reflection Quote: "With awareness brings health, healing, and longevity. I felt like I did not belong, but I persevered anyway. And to my delight, I began to love myself."

INTRODUCTION

Unconscious biases are stereotypes or prejudgments made by others about an identified group of people. These stereotypes and prejudgments are not often based on factual information and have a distinct tendency to be founded upon limited societal images and interactions with others that are skewed. Hence, our social context impacts our reality in our interactions with one another.

Rogers and Nesbitt (2020) note that is it important in health care for patients to feel that they are both seen and heard by their providers. Health care workers' and providers' failure to recognize, listen to, and respect all patients in interactions can result in distrust. When patients distrust health care workers and providers, they will have difficulty engaging in treatment and following health care recommendations. This means poor compliance and worsening of symptoms of disease, illnesses, or syndromes.

Rogers and Nesbitt (2020), both physicians, in addressing unconscious biases in obstetrics and gynecology office practices, discussed how racism is at the core of the problem of health disparities. For example, the false belief that Black people are resistant to pain and injury has historically led to doctors undertreating their pain (Badreldin et al, 2109; Hoffman et al., 2016; Lee et al., 2019). The maternal mortality and morbidity rate for Black women is three to four times higher than that of White women in the US (Black Maternal Health Caucus, 2020; Howell, 2018). Black women are less likely to have the same level of surgical intervention that White women receive, and they are more likely to undergo a hysterectomy related to cervical and endometrial cancer

(Temkin et al., 2018). The latter cancer-related statistics were attributed to low SES, being underinsured, having other comorbidities, and loss to follow-up. Rogers and Nesbitt (2020) noted five take-aways in overcoming racism and unconscious bias in office practice settings (in particular, in obstetrics and gynecology office practice):

1. Racism is a continuing problem in health care.
2. Physicians must acknowledge their role and commit to working for equality.
3. There are racial disparities in pain management, cancer treatment, and maternal mortality.
4. If you witness micro-inequities in the office, they should be addressed.
5. The office staff are representatives of the physician; if they do not make a Black patient feel welcome, it can negatively affect the patient's relationship with the physician. (Rogers & Nesbitt, 2020)

Clendon (2020) noted the historical origins of unconscious bias in social psychology and the cognitive sciences. However, **implicit or unconscious biases** are an automatic response, as the human brain quickly makes judgments about situations and people that are solely based upon a person's environment, life experiences, and background (Mahzarin et al., 2013). Humans prefer persons that they can identify with physically and who come from backgrounds similar to their own.

Unconscious biases interfere with one's ability to recognize when a person who looks differently than themselves, shares a good idea, that they disregard what the other person says as having no value; choosing not to listen. Hence, the ability to make objective decisions is impaired (Clendon, 2020). According to Wilkerson and Kirkwood (2018), training to identify unconscious biases in organizations can bring awareness to unfounded and false judgments of others. Over time, training can create environments where unconscious and implicit biases are not tolerated.

PERCEIVED DISCRIMINATION

Perceived discrimination is the belief that different treatment and interactions are the negative result of a group a person belongs to; for minorities, this may be the racial or ethnic group with which they identify. However, perceived discrimination can also be attributed to socioeconomics, mental health, disability, education, gender, religion, and developmental stages, among many other aspects of being human.

Perceived Discrimination and Mental Health

Having a mental illness can be isolating, as affected individuals struggle to manage the signs and symptoms of their illness while functioning daily in families and communities that may not understand their challenges. The stigmatization of mental health in itself can lead to unaffected persons having perceptions of the mentally ill as a group to which they do not belong (Bagci et al., 2018). **In-group identification** relates to solidarity and how persons with a common issue cope positively or negatively with their identified concern. For persons with mental health issues, societal views of their presenting symptomatology are correlated with perceived discrimination.

Worldwide, people with mental illness may encounter issues such as homelessness, unemployment, challenges with the completion of education, hunger, poor access to quality health care related to either having no insurance or being underinsured, and poverty (Filmer, 2008; Mizunoya, 2013; Bagci et al., 2018). In 2019, it was estimated that during the month of January, 17 out of every 10,000 people in the US were homeless on a single night (National Alliance to End Homelessness, 2020a). This means that, nationally, 567,715 people of different genders, families with children, single people, adolescents, and people of different races and cultural backgrounds were homeless. Fifteen percent of the homeless population have chronic medical issues, chronic substance use disorders, and a serious mental illness (National Alliance to End Homelessness, 2020a; National Alliance to End Homelessness, 2020b).

PSYCHOLOGICAL WELL-BEING IN ETHNIC-MINORITY ADOLESCENTS

Stevens and Thijs (2018) examined the relationship between psychological well-being and perceived group discrimination in a study conducted in the Netherlands. The participants were 354 Moroccan-Dutch adolescents who were interviewed and asked to identify situations in which they felt discriminated against. Eleven percent answered that they had experienced personal discrimination by the police and in school; approximately 1.5% stated they had experienced discrimination in shops and on the street. Overall, the results of the study found that there was a correlation between perceived group discrimination when the adolescents and their parents externalized problems with aggression and anger, and internalized worries and fears. The latter did not impact personal self-esteem. However, Stevens and Thijs (2018) did find that perceived personal discrimination was negatively associated with the personal self-esteem of the adolescents.

Adolescents who had a strong ethnic group identification did not (nor did their parents) internalize problems, nor was perceived group discrimination a concern. However, when adolescents and their parents had a weak ethnic group identification, problems were internalized and perceived discrimination was identified. Stevens and Thijs (2018) found that personal self-esteem and perceived group discrimination were unrelated. However, members of a minority group can be impacted negatively by discrimination, even if they do not personally experience it themselves.

Generalized Anxiety and Depression Among Muslim American College Students

There are approximately 1.8 billion Muslims worldwide and 2.3 billion Christians (Pew Research, 2019). Current estimates are that the US, by 2060, will remain a predominantly Christian country (Pew Research, 2019). Muslims in the US are diverse in their backgrounds with regard to religious practices, race, and country of origin (Sirin & Fine, 2008). Since the September 11 terrorist attacks, Muslim-Americans have experienced hate crimes and discrimination. For example, in 2018, 14.6% of the 1,617 anti-religious hate crimes committed in the US were identified as involving victims of anti-Islamic (Muslim) bias (Federal Bureau of Investigation, 2018). Comparatively, the highest percentage of anti-religious hate crimes (56.9%) involved anti-Jewish bias. Anti-Islamic crimes were rated second (Federal Bureau of Investigation, 2018).

Lowe et al. (2018) conducted a study of 141 Muslim American college students at Montclair State University in New Jersey. The findings indicated that there was a positive correlation between perceived discrimination and generalized anxiety disorder (GAD) and major depression. Lowe et al. (2018) used the Patient Health Questionnaire-8 (PHQ-8; Kroenke et al., 2001) to assess for major depression symptoms, and the GAD-7 (Spitzer et al., 2006) to assess for symptoms of GAD. Perceived discrimination was measured using the General Ethnic Discrimination Scale, which has been shown to be valid and reliable when used with Asian, White, Black, and Latinx persons. The results indicated that the Muslim American college students had a significant risk for developing major depression and general anxiety of 42.9%. It was also noted that Muslim American college students who had a strong Muslim group identity were more likely to experience GAD.

In-group identification can bring about unity and even a sense of purpose, as people with similarities bond and provide support to one another. Hence, in-group identification can be protective for persons experiencing perceived discrimination. However, when the identity of the group has strong cultural, racial, and religious similarities, discrimination is still likely to occur because the group's physical characteristics related to biological factors and their desire to maintain customs and religious traditions can make them easily recognizable. In the latter case, attempts to assimilate and adapt to the dominant culture can prove futile. Discriminatory acts may continue to occur despite the in-group identification.

SUICIDE IN THE U.S.

In the US, during the years 1999 through 2018, suicide was the tenth leading cause of death, with a total of 48,344 Americans succumbing (CDC, 2020). Causes of death by suicide were classified into 11 categories: Unspecified (n= 91, 0.2%), other specified and not elsewhere classifiable (n = 103, 0.2%), transportation related (n = 190, 0.4%), fire/burn (n = 214, 0.4%), drowning (n = 522, 1.1%), other specified and classifiable (n = 669, 1.4%), cut/pierce (n = 897, 1.9%), fall (n= 1,149, 2.4%), poisoning (n = 6,237, 12.9%), suffocation (n = 13,840, 28.6%), and firearms (n = 24,432, 50.5%). These data not only include all age groups, but also both sexes and all races and ethnicities (CDC, 2018). Suicide correlates with depression, emotional pain, and isolation. All human beings suffer with the latter. However, discrimination and health disparities associated with mental illness may increase the likelihood of self-harm.

Mental Health Among American Indians and Alaska Natives

The second leading cause of death for American Indians and Alaska Natives aged 10–34 years in 2017 was suicide. More members of this group reported experiencing psychological distress within the 30 days prior to being asked (9.2% of those surveyed) than were non-Hispanic Whites (3.7% of those surveyed; CDC, 2018; US DHHS, Office of Minority Health, 2019a). Within the second decade of life, 75% of American Indians and Alaska Natives were more likely to suffer unintentional injuries, suicide, homicide, and violent deaths than non-Hispanic Whites. For adult American Indians and Alaska Natives aged 18 years and older who were diagnosed with a major depressive episode, 61.2% received treatment in 2018; meanwhile, 68.5% of non-Hispanic Whites received treatment during the same year. The death rate from suicide for American Indians and Alaska Natives is 20% higher than for non-Hispanic Whites. Adolescent females of American Indian and Alaska Native ancestry between the ages of 15 and 19 years are three times more likely than non-Hispanic White females of the same age to die from mental- and behavioral-health-related causes (Substance Abuse and Mental Health Services Administration [SAMHSA], 2019; CDC, 2019a).

African Americans and Mental Health in America

During the years 1980 through 1995, rates of suicide among African American children and adolescents aged 10–14 years increased by 233%. Among non-Hispanic Whites, that increase was 120%. African American females in grades 9 through 12, in comparison to non-white Hispanic females, were 70% more likely to attempt acts of self-harm via suicide (US DHHS, Office of Minority Health, 2019c).

For African American men (11.4%), death by suicide in 2017 was four times greater than that among African American women (2.8%). For African Americans aged 15–24 years, death by suicide was the second leading cause of death (CDC, 2019a; US DHHS, Office of Minority Health, 2019c). However, non-Hispanic White males (28.2%) and females (7.9%) have higher rates of suicide when compared to other racial groups (CDC, 2019b; US DHHS, Office of Minority Health, 2019c).

Asian Americans and Pacific Islanders and Mental Health

According to the American Psychiatric Association (2020), suicide was the leading cause of death in 2017 for Asian Americans aged 15–24 years (CDC, 2019a). In comparison to non-Hispanic Whites, Asian Americans' suicide rate is nearly half that for females (Asian Americans, 3.9; non-Hispanic Whites, 7.9) and males (Asian Americans, 9.9; non-Hispanic Whites, 28.2). Approximately 2.7 million Asian Americans and Pacific Islanders have been diagnosed with a mental illness or substance use disorder (SAMHSA, 2018). However, comparatively, Asian Americans (substance use, 4.8%; alcohol use 3.8%) have lower alcohol and substance use than other minority groups and non-Hispanic Whites (substance use 7.4%; alcohol use 14.7%) in the US (SAMHSA, 2018).

The diagnosis of posttraumatic stress disorder (PTSD) associated with immigrating from Southeast Asia to the US was noted to occur among 70% of Southeast Asian refugees who sought mental health treatment (NIH, 2006). Asian Americans and Pacific Islanders are three times less likely than non-Hispanic Whites to seek mental health services because of the limited cultural and linguistic competencies of health care providers (APA, 2020; US DHHS, Office of Minority Health, 2019b).

Latinx Communities and Mental Health

Socioeconomic status (SES) significantly impacts the mental health of Lantinx who live below the poverty level. While the suicide rate for Hispanics is less than half that of non-Hispanic Whites, Hispanic men (11.2) are four times more likely to harm themselves than are Hispanic women (2.6). During the year 2017, for Hispanics aged 15–34 years, suicide was the second leading cause of death. Between 2015 and 2016, 3.7% of Hispanics over the age of 18 years reported experiencing psychological distress over a period of 30 days, the same percentage as non-Hispanic Whites (CDC, 2019; US DHHS, Office of Minority Health, 2019a).

THE SOCIOECONOMICS OF MENTAL HEALTH

Living below the poverty level was noted to be a potential contributing factor for increases in psychological distress. Upon review of poverty statistics by race, at this time, Blacks in the US have the highest rate of poverty, with 20.8% of African Americans living below the federal poverty level. Hispanics have a poverty rate of 17.6%, Asians 10.1%, and White, non-Hispanics 8.1% (US Census Bureau, 2019). The median income for families during 2018 was $63,179. Annual household income in 2018 was $51,450 for Hispanics, $70, 642 for non-Hispanic Whites, $41,361 for Blacks, and $87,194 for Asians (US Census Bureau, 2019).

Low-Income Immigrant Children and Health Insurance Coverage

Jarlenski et al. (2016) reviewed data from the National Survey of Children's Health beginning in 2003 (Blumberg et al., 2005) and running through 2012 (National Center for Health Statistics, 2017). The data included 83,612 children within families that had incomes less than 200% of the federal poverty level. The ages of the children were between 0 and 17 years. Three immigration statuses were used to categorize the children: (1) immigrant children, (2) citizen children with nonimmigrant parents, and (3) citizen children with immigrant parents. Multivariable regression analysis was applied to control for the children's access to care and health insurance coverage. The findings showed that, in all three of the immigration groups, from 2003 through 2012, gains were made in access to care and health insurance coverage. While immigrant children still have lower insurance coverage, the US has increased access to a primary health care provider, which maintains consistency in care received. Hence, given the lower incomes of immigrant children, they too are at high risk for psychological distress associated with poverty.

Low-Income Postpartum Women and Allostatic Load

McEwen (2005) noted that the adaptive processes by which the human body maintains a state of homeostasis is by producing chemical messengers, such as cortisol and adrenaline to mediate stress. However, as the body is subjected repeatedly to stress and stressors, the adaptive response no longer is effective in protecting the body. Hence, the body becomes more susceptible to disease (and injury). This process is referred to as the allostatic load (AL).

The AL was assessed among 2,448 postpartum women who were enrolled in the Eunice Kennedy Shriver National Institute for Child Health and Human Development Community Child Health Network. The women were Latina, White, and African Amcrican, and belonged primarily to low-income families. The women's infants were all live births at greater than or equal to 20 weeks gestation. Shalowitz et al. (2019) followed the women over 12 months, measuring their AL. The AL was measured by blood pressure, diurnal cortisol slope, hemoglobin A1C, body mass index, high-sensitive C-reactive protein, waist: hip ratio, and total cholesterol and high-density lipoproteins.

African American women were found to have significantly greater AL-associated health risks in comparison to their White and Latina counterparts. For White women, breastfeeding was protective. However, for women who experienced pregnancy-related complications, their AL was higher during the first year of the study. With an elevated AL during the first year, health disparities either worsened or remained unchanged. Shalowitz et al. (2019) noted that AL profiles were present in White, African American, and Latina women from the birth of their infant to age one year, and that health disparities did not improve; breastfeeding was the primary protective factor identified.

Black Women and Death in Childbirth

Maternal deaths are those that occur while a woman is pregnant or up to 42 days after a pregnancy has been terminated, in absence of an incident or accident contributing to the mother's death (CDC, 2020). Maternal mortality continues to increase within the US, with Black women experiencing death rates 3–4 times higher than those of White women. Pregnancy-related deaths for White women are 14.7 out of 100,000 live births; for Black women, the value is 37.1 out of 100,000 live births, and for Latinas, it is 11.8 out of 100,000 live births (CDC, 2020). The National Center for Health Statistics first released data to the public in 2007; these data show the health disparities impacting Black women and the high rate of maternal deaths for this group. Small et al. (2017) describe the high rates of maternal deaths among African American women as a public health inequity. It is imperative that nationally representative longitudinal studies be conducted that follow Black women over the course of their pregnancies to identify risk factors that can be addressed to promote health and deter death during and after pregnancy.

Chronic Pain and Nonpharmacologic Treatment Access

Opioid abuse costs the US an estimated $78.5 billion a year. It contributes to increased financial burdens in addiction treatment, the criminal justice system, loss of productivity in the workplace, and healthcare costs. In 2018, an average of 128 Americans died each day of an overdose of synthetic opioids (i.e., fentanyl), prescription pain relievers, or heroin (National Institute on Drug Abuse, 2020).

Opioid abuse has been identified as a national crisis in the US. However, poor access by low-income racial and ethnic minorities to nonpharmacologic treatments for chronic pain is common (Cheng et al., 2019). A study by Cheng et al. (2019) used both qualitative and quantitative methods while applying the Science Café methodology. An event was held in an urban community center in Boston, Massachusetts, as a means to elicit volunteers. Audio and video recordings were used to obtain data from focus groups, as were self-reported questionnaires. Thirty study participants self-identified as either health care providers (54%) or patients (46%) experiencing chronic pain. Nineteen percent of participants were Latinx, 42% were Black, and 77% identified as female. Participants' average age was 45 years.

Cheng et al. (2019) noted three themes in their study results: (1) both patients and providers value the patient–provider relationship and acknowledge the need for better communication with patients who suffer from chronic pain; (2) nonpharmacologic options for chronic pain management are warranted; and (3) larger sociodemographic and contextual factors influence the management of chronic pain. The need for additional research on barriers to accessing nonpharmacologic chronic pain treatments was indicated. This is a health disparity because, if racially and ethnically diverse populations are not educated on nonpharmacologic alternative treatments in the management of chronic pain, they may be at higher risk for engaging in opioid misuse, given that approximately 80% of persons who use heroin were first prescribed opioids by a health care provider (National Institute on Drug Abuse, 2020).

HEALTH CARE FOR LESBIAN, GAY, BISEXUAL, AND TRANSGENDER PEOPLE

Historically, the ability to identify as a lesbian, gay, bisexual, or transgender (LGBT) person in America was not included in the US Census (US Census Bureau, 2020). These categories were used for the first time in the 2020 Census. However, six national data systems have collected sexual orientation data for over ten years. These systems are the American Community Survey, Youth Risk Behavior Survey, National Crime Victimization Survey, National Survey of Family Growth, National Health and Nutrition and Examination Survey, and Behavioral Risk Factor Surveillance Survey. Additionally, the National Health Interview Survey and the National Survey of Drug Use and Health were both used to collect sexual orientation data in 2013 and 2015, respectively (ODPHP, 2020).

LGBT persons come from different socioeconomic spheres and represent different ethnicities, races, and religions. Notably, in 2010, the US Healthy People Initiative issued a companion document that discussed the lack of substantial data to formalize a plan to address health care disparities within the LGBT community. As a result, data have gradually been gathered by select health organizations and agencies so that health disparities can be accurately identified.

LGBT Discrimination

Transphobia, **biphobia**, and **homophobia** are terminologies used to define the confusion, frustration, and discriminatory acts that heterosexuals perpetrate against the LGBT community. A **phobia** is a fear that perpetuates an irrational reaction or behavior that manifests as intense anxiety. In the American Psychiatric Association's Diagnostic Criteria from the DSM-5 (2013), phobias are described as:

A. Marked fear or anxiety about a specific object or situation (e.g., flying, heights, animals, receiving an injection, seeing blood). Note: In children, the fear or anxiety may be expressed by crying, tantrums, freezing, or clinging.

B. The phobic object or situation almost always provokes immediate fear or anxiety.

C. The phobic object or situation is actively avoided or endured with intense fear or anxiety.

D. The fear or anxiety is out of proportion to the actual danger posed by the specific object or situation and to the sociocultural context.

E. The fear, anxiety, or avoidance is persistent, typically lasting for six months or more.

F. The fear, anxiety, or avoidance causes clinically significant distress or impairment in social, occupational, or other important areas of functioning.

G. The disturbance is not better explained by the symptoms of another mental disorder, including fear, anxiety, and avoidance of situations associated with panic-like symptoms or other incapacitating symptoms (as in agoraphobia);

objects or situations related to obsessions (as in posttraumatic stress disorder); separation from home or attachment figures (as in separation anxiety disorder). (American Psychiatric Association, 2013, pp. 116–117)

The concept of **fear** involves that which constitutes a misunderstanding or misinterpretation of a person(s) or situation that, taken out of context, leads to discriminatory acts. On February 25, 2021, the US House of Representatives passed the Equality Act. If also passed by the Senate and signed by the President of the United States, this bill would prohibit discrimination against individuals based on their gender identity, sexual orientation, and sex. Protected areas would include housing, the jury system, federal funding, education, employment, and public facilities and accommodations. In addition, the Department of Justice would be allowed to intervene within the federal court system to address issues related to gender identity and sexual orientation (Congress.gov, 2020; Human Rights Campaign, 2021).

The discrimination committed against the LGBT community significantly affects their health. LGBT persons with health issues are more likely to present to the healthcare system late in a disease process, are unlikely to trust the healthcare system, and, as a result, may not follow up with care or maintain continuity of care. LGBT persons are also more likely to have poor levels of health care provided while engaged in treatment (Glasper, 2016).

Women's Health and the LGBT Community

Heterosexual women are more likely to have better health outcomes than women who identify as bisexual, queer (same-gender-loving or pansexual), or lesbian (Mosack et al., 2103). Obesity, cardiovascular disease, alcoholism, and smoking (Cochran, 2001; Drabble & Trocki, 2005; Gruskin & Gorden, 2006) are all health deviations and risk factors that impact the mortality and morbidity of women who identify as LBQ (lesbian, bisexual, or queer). Bisexual and lesbian women who classified themselves as either *femme* or *butch*, according to Hiestand et al. (2007), have different experiences when seeking health care. Women who self-identified as being *butch* reported receiving poor health care treatment and fewer gynecological examinations than women who self-identified as *femme*.

Bisexual and lesbian women are least likely to maintain a pattern of screenings for women's health, such as annual physical examinations, tests for sexually transmitted infections, and Pap smears (Agenor et al., 2015; Charlton et al., 2011). Johnson and Nemeth (2014) conducted a grounded theory study to examine health disparities among bisexual and lesbian women. Forty-five students were recruited from universities in the southwest US. Criteria for inclusion were women between the ages of 18 and 24 years who self-identified as queer, lesbian, or bisexual. Of the 45 study participants, four were bisexual, one was transgender, and—with the exception of one Latinx and one Asian participant—all participants were White.

Johnson and Nemeth (2014) conducted interviews with each study participant about their experiences in health care. An explanatory framework was utilized and was divided into three phases: pre-interaction (expectations and seeking of health care), health care interaction (disclosure of sexual orientation and moment of truth; provider attributes were knowledge, communication, and attitudes), and outcomes (health outcomes and proximal outcomes; knowledge-seeking behavior, health-seeking behavior, disguise sexual orientation, change provider, and others). Participants reported that their conversations with health care providers were at times antagonistic, particularly when discussing birth control; providers would inquire about a woman's sexual preference and ask if they would be returning to a same-sex relationship or maintain a heterosexual relationship (Johnson & Nemeth, 2014). This antagonistic question by the healthcare providers, was likely related to inquiry about prescribing birth control. However, was disrespectful nonetheless.

Full disclosure of health deviations and sexual history is imperative for preventive care and disease management. When lesbian and bisexual women do not feel comfortable disclosing their health problems to health care providers they perceive to be judgmental, they may be less likely to engage in preventive visits, thus increasing their risk for late diagnoses of disease processes (e.g., cancer).

Transgender, Genderqueer, and Cisgender Health Disparities

Lefevor et al.(2019) examined the health disparities between cisgender, genderqueer (nonbinary; neither traditionally female or male), and transgender persons as an extension of minority stress theory. A sample of 3,568 college students from the Collegiate Mental Health's 2012–2016 database were selected, with 892 students identifying as being outside the gender binary, and 892 identifying as transgender women or men. Analyses were conducted of outcome measures and demographics acquired during the participants' first counseling session. The findings revealed that college students who identified as genderqueer experienced more traumatic events in their lives than those who identified as transgender or cisgender. Fifty percent of genderqueer individuals reported experiencing traumatic events. Genderqueer individuals also reported having been sexually abused and harassed.

Suicidality and self-harm were prevalent in genderqueer individuals. Approximately two-thirds of college students who identified as genderqueer had suicidal ideation, and nearly 50% had tried to harm themselves (Lefevor et al., 2019). In comparison to transgender and cisgender individuals, more genderqueer students had eating concerns, depression, psychological distress, and anxiety. Systemic discrimination, poor access to medical and legal services, and the lack of knowledge of others about persons who identify as genderqueer contributed to their stress as a minority group (Hendricks & Testa, 2012; Lefevor et al., 2019; Meyer 2001).

PSYCHOLOGICAL IMPLICATIONS FOR HEALTH DISPARITIES

Psychologically, when perceived discrimination is experienced by people seeking health care, an immediate distrust of the health care provider or workers with whom the negative communication or actions occurred, can cause affected persons to withdraw and become angry, depressed, anxious, or frustrated. Hausmann et al. (2011) conducted a study on the impacts of perceived discrimination in health care on patient and provider communication. Participants in the study were 253 White patients and 100 African American patients being treated for osteoarthritis in two Veterans Affairs healthcare systems. Additionally, 63 orthopedic surgeons were recruited to participate in the study.

Criteria for the patients to participate were that they had chronic hip or knee pain, had no history of joint replacement surgery, were aged 50 years or older, and did not have a diagnosis suggestive of an inflammatory arthritis. The orthopedic surgeons providing care to the patients were first-year general surgery residents or residents in their second to sixth year of orthopedic residency at one of the two participating clinics. Areas measured that could impact patients' experiences with communication and discrimination included self-identified race (non-Hispanic White and non-Hispanic African American), highest educational attainment (high school or less), previous visits to the orthopedic clinic, age, quality of life (SF-12 Scale with physical and mental components), and annual income (missing, less than \$20,000, or greater than or less than \$20,000) (Hausmann et al., 2011; Ware et al., 1996).

An observational cross-sectional study was used by Hausmann et al. (2011). The groups of White and African American patients were surveyed about their experiences with classism and racism they had encountered within the healthcare system in the past. The surveys were completed prior to a clinic visit within the Veterans Affairs health system. Then, the clinic visits between the health care providers and the patients were audio recorded. The audio recordings were coded for affective, nonverbal affective tone, and instrumental communication content, such as patient engagement/activation, rapport building, psychosocial exchange, and biomedical exchange. Participants were asked to rate their clinic visits based on the ease of communicating with the provider, provider respectfulness/warmth, and informativeness of the visit. Additionally, regression models were stratified by patients' race and used to assess the relationship of classism and racism with outcomes in communication (Hausmann et al., 2011). The Everyday Discrimination Scale was used to assess the frequency with which a person was treated unfairly based on their socioeconomic class/status and race. These scales have Cronbach's alphas of 0.93 and 0.90 for racism and classism, respectively (Williams et al., 2008).

The results of the Hausmann et al. (2011) study found that African American patients had higher levels of perceived classism and racism than their White counterparts. While 26% of White patients reported experiencing racism, 70% of African Americans did. For classism, 53% of Whites experienced classism, as did 73% of African Americans. Higher levels of perceived racism were noted to be associated with providers and African American patients having a decreased ease of communication (odds ration [OR] = 0.22, 95% confidence interval [CI] = 0.07, 0.67), low level of provider warmth/respectfulness (OR = 0.19, 95% CI = 0.05, 0.72), and less positive nonverbal affect by providers (Beta = −0.34, 95% CI = −0.66, −0.01) and patients (Beta = −0.41, 95% CI = −0.73, −0.09). The results for perceived classism were similar (Hausmann et al., 2011).

For White patients, less psychosocial communication (Beta = 4.18, 95% CI = −7.68, −0.68) was associated with perceived racism, ease of communication (OR = 0.43, 95% CI = 0.20, 0.89), and low patient ratings of clinic visit informativeness (OR = 0.40, 95% CI = 0.23, 0.71). The results of perceived classism were again similar (Hausmann et al., 2011). The Hausmann et al. (2011) results concluded that the pervasive impact of perceived discrimination in healthcare settings can negatively impact patient–provider communication and nonverbal affective communication with African American patients. The latter can have long-term effects on African American patients' willingness to interface with healthcare systems because of these negative experiences. It is recommended that training programs be developed for health care providers to increase provider awareness of the effects that discrimination has on patient–provider relationships.

LANGUAGE BARRIERS

Spanish-speaking patients who present to emergency departments within the US may encounter staff who speak English to them or health care workers and providers who speak Spanish with varied levels of proficiency, according to Benda et al. (2019) and Showstack (2019). The Patient Protection and Affordable Care Act (ACA, see Chapter 1), enacted in 2010, is a healthcare reform law that was designed to support innovations in medical care that can decrease the cost of health care delivery, and increase the number of insured by expanding the Medicaid program and providing federal subsidies to lower-income Americans to help them afford insurance premiums (ACA, 2010). Current health care innovations related to language include technologies, such as translator phones at the patient's bedside, that assist with language translation, and computerized electronic devices connecting healthcare systems to translators available 24-hours a day and covering a variety of languages and dialects. Additionally, health care facilities receiving federal funding from the US government (ACA, 2010) are required to offer patients an interpreter when they enter the facility for care. Hence, either an in-person certified speaker of the language, a translator via a phone call, or a computer-based video live translator must be provided. Failure to do so is a violation of the law.

Culture and Language Barriers

Patriksson et al. (2019) conducted a field study applying a hermeneutic lifeworld approach, interviews with healthcare professionals and parents, and participant observation in their examination of conditions impacting communication between parents on a neonatal ward and health care professionals facing language barriers. Three neonatal units, including one that was a neonatal intensive care unit, were within the same Swedish region, and the three hospitals collaborated with each other in care delivery. Unit 1 had 130 healthcare professionals and 23 patient beds; Unit 2 had 48 healthcare professionals and 11 patient beds; and Unit 3 had 51 healthcare professionals and 12 patient beds. The length of stay for hospitalizations varied from 8.2, to 8.4, and 14.2 days, respectively (Patriksson et al., 2019).

Patriksson et al. (2019) collected data about the ways that language barriers affect communications between health care professionals and patients over three months in 2018. The study encompassed 62 field hours, 20 interviews with health care professionals, 52 observations, and ten patient interviews during day, evening, and night shifts. The parents were immigrants from various countries. Hence, a variation in race and culture shaped approaches to education on breastfeeding and parents' gender roles in communicating information. The results showed that parents who could speak English preferred to use English to speak with their health care professionals. However, the health care professionals preferred to use an interpreter out of concern that the parents would not understand the information provided to them about the care of their neonate. Both parties were frustrated, as the parents would request a family member who spoke English to translate if needed, while health care professionals preferred an interpreter. Interestingly, parents preferred a multilingual health care professional who not only understood their language, but to whom they could also culturally relate.

American Sign Language

Hommes et al. (2018) examined the perceptions of American Sign Language interpreters to barriers to healthcare communication in hard-of-hearing and deaf patients. A ten-item survey consisting of Likert scales, open-ended, and multiple-choice questions was given to 146 conference attendees at the National Symposium of Healthcare Interpreting in 2015. Approximately 25% of attendees responded, with 81% sharing that health care providers "hardly ever use teach-back methods" (Hommes et al., 2018, p. 956); as a result, there is no way to determine if patients that are deaf or hard of hearing understand the information that was taught to them. This places these patients at risk for medication errors, with prescribed medications being self-administered at home, or procedural errors, such as a patient changing their post-operative dressing at home. These behaviors by health care providers contribute to health disparities in this population.

Healthcare facilities, according to Hommes et al. (2018), should be accountable for health literacy, empowerment of patients, ensuring that their facility is staffed with American Sign Language interpreters, and improving communication among health care professionals and their patients with hearing impairments. Hearing-impaired patients come from various races and cultures; the commonality for those who use American Sign Language is their communication technique. Therefore, it is imperative that sign language interpreters be present for this population to ensure that information is conveyed for timely health screenings (i.e., breast mammography, testicular self-examinations, etc.), health procedures, informed consent for surgeries, and the safe self-administration of prescribed medications.

Injustices in Health Care

When healthcare organizations fail to provide linguistic services to patients with language barriers, this constitutes an epistemic injustice (Peled, 2016). With worldwide immigration, healthcare organizations are obligated to serve the needs of all people. Health care disparities can only be addressed when barriers to health care delivery are alleviated. Therefore, for timely, accurate, and quality patient-centered care to be delivered, health care professionals must use interpreters and/or devices that facilitate the interpretation of patients' native language.

SUMMARY

Experiencing health disparities involving humans of different genders, races, religions, cultures, abilities, and socioeconomic backgrounds can be emotionally damaging. Trust between health care professionals and patients is affected when patients perceive that their very existence is not valued and that their health care will be suboptimal because they are different. Diversity is a normal occurrence within the human species. Maltreatment by health care workers and providers can impact patient outcomes.

Unconscious and implicit biases, when brought to the awareness of health care workers and providers, can result in the eradication of these practices. However, organizations must commit to educating their health care workers and providers. Overt and perceived discrimination is detrimental to the health and well-being of those affected. For health care disparities perpetuated by health care workers and providers to be eliminated, training must be required.

Moreover, health care organizations should be met with fines when there is a failure to hold staff accountable. After all, human lives are priceless.

UNDERSTANDING UNCONSCIOUS BIAS AND PERCEIVED DISCRIMINATION WITHIN HEALTH DISPARITIES

Directions: Read each question or statement and discuss how implicit and unconscious biases impact persons of low income, racial and ethnic minorities, persons with mental illness, and persons with language barriers. Discuss how perceived discrimination affects vulnerable populations.

1. What is implicit or unconscious bias?
2. How does implicit or unconscious bias impact people?
3. Should healthcare organizations provide training to health care workers and providers on the topics of implicit or unconscious biases? Why?
4. Explain what perceived discrimination is and why it occurs.
5. Identify human characteristics and differences that may lead to discrimination by fellow humans.
6. Psychological damage can be incurred when someone is isolated and treated as if they do not exist. **Consider this:** Have you ever intentionally ignored someone because you were afraid of them or appalled by their physical presentation related to learned stereotypes?
7. What makes one human life of more value than another?
8. Should health care be a privilege granted to all persons? If yes, why? If no, who should make the decision to distribute health care to diverse groups of people?
9. Does systemic racism contribute to health care disparities?
10. How do religious differences contribute to group discrimination?
11. Do hate crimes regularly occur within the US?
12. Provide an example of in-group pride and self-esteem.
13. How does poverty impact mental health?
14. How does poverty associated with underinsurance cause physiological complications?
15. Can stress experienced by identified minority groups lead to psychological problems?
16. Can healthcare environments be changed to create a climate of acceptance and respect? If yes, who is in charge of implementing this change?

CASE STUDY: SILENCE

I sit in my hospital room watching the nurses and staff walk by. I would love for someone to talk to me. I read lips, but sometimes it takes me time. See, I am newly deaf and, while my sign language is very good, reading lips can be difficult. I noticed that, because not all the staff know American Sign Language, my room is avoided. I may get a quick smile or nod, which I appreciate, but that is it. I wonder, is this how people who have a language barrier get treated because they do not speak English?

Discussion: Can the person who uses American Sign Language have the same language barrier experience as a person who does not speak English?

Figure 1. Effective communication

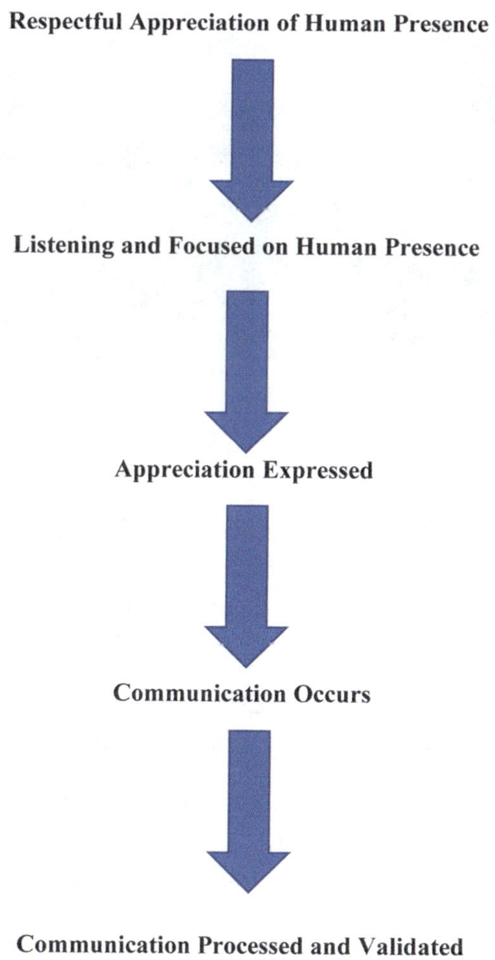

Figure 2. Fallen and submerged

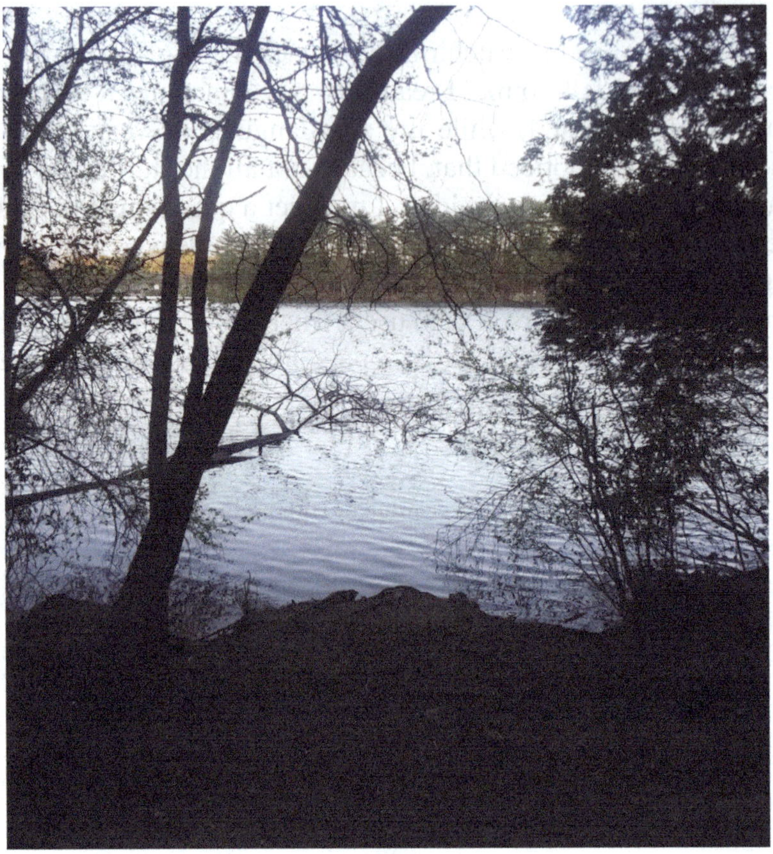

REFERENCES

Agénor, M., Bailey, Z., Krieger, N., & Bryn, S. (2015). Exploring the cervical cancer screening experiences of Black Lesbian, Bisexual, and Queer women: The role of patient-provider communication. *Women & Health*, *55*(6), 717–736. doi:10.1080/03630242.2015.1039182 PMID:25909663

American Psychiatric Association. (2013). *Desk reference to the diagnostic criteria from DSM-5*. American Psychiatric Association.

American Psychiatric Association. (2020). *Mental health facts for Asian Americans/Pacific Islanders*. https://www.psychiatry.org/psychiatrists/cultural-competency/education/asian-american-patients

Badreldin, N., Grobman, W. A., & Yee, L. M. (2019). Racial disparities in postpartum pain management. *Obstetrics and Gynecology*, *134*(6), 1147–1153. doi:10.1097/AOG.0000000000003561 PMID:31764723

Bagci, S. C., Turnuklu, A., & Bekezci, E. (2018). The buffering role of in-group identification and intergroup on the association between perceived discrimination and mental health. *Applied Social Psychology*, *28*(5), 293–305. doi:10.1002/casp.2357

Benda, N. C., Fairbanks, R. J., Higginbotham, D. J., & Bisantz, L. L. A. M. (2019). Observational study to understand interpreter service use in emergency medicine: Why the key may lie outside of the initial provider assessment. *Emergency Medicine Journal*, *36*(10), 582–588. doi:10.1136/emermed-2019-208420 PMID:31320333

Black Maternal Health Caucus. (2020). *About the Black Maternal Health Momnibus Act of 2020*. https://blackmaternalhealthcaucus-underwood.house.gov/Momnibus

Blumberg, S. J., Olson, L., Frankel, M. R., Osborn, L., Srinath, K. P., & Giambo, P. (2005). Design and operation of the National Survey of Children's Health, 2003. *Vital and Health Statistics. Series 1, Programs and Collection Procedures*, (43), 1–131. https://pubmed.ncbi.nlm.nih.gov/25078122/ PMID:25078122

Centers for Disease Control and Prevention. (2018). *Health, United States, 2017: With special feature on mortality*. https://www.cdc.gov/nchs/data/hus/hus17.pdf

Centers for Disease Control and Prevention. (2019a). *National Vital Statistics Report, 68*(9). Table 10. https://www.cdc.gov/nchs/data/nvsr/nvsr68/nvsr68_09.pdf

Centers for Disease Control and Prevention. (2019b). *Injury prevention and control: WISQARS injury data*. https://www.cdc.gov/injury/wisqars/index.html

Centers for Disease Control and Prevention. (2020). *WISQARS-Leading cause of death reports, 1981–2018*. https://webappa.cdc.gov/cgi-bin/broker.exe

Centers for Disease Control and Prevention, National Center for Health Statistics. (2020). *First data released on maternal mortality in over a decade.* https://www.cdc.gov/nchs/pressroom/nchs_press_releases/2020/202001_MMR.htm

Centers for Disease Control and Prevention, National Center for Injury Prevention and Control. (2018). *United States suicide data, 2018.* https://www.cdc.gov/mmwr/volumes/70/wr/mm7008a1.htm

Charlton, B. M., Corliss, H. L., Missmer, S. A., Frazier, A. L., Rosario, M., Kahn, J. A., & Austin, S. B. (2011). Reproductive health screening disparities and sexual orientation in a cohort study of U.S. adolescent and young adult females. *The Journal of Adolescent Health, 49*(5), 505–510. doi:10.1016/j.jadohealth.2011.03.013 PMID:22018565

Cheng, T., D'Amico, S., Luo, M., Lestoquoy, A. S., Yinusa-Nyahkoon, L., Laird, L. D., & Gardiner, P. M. (2019). Health disparities in access to nonpharmacologic therapies in an urban community. *Journal of Alternative and Complementary Medicine (New York, N.Y.), 25*(1), 48–60. doi:10.1089/acm.2018.0217

Cochran, S. D. (2001). Emerging issues in research on lesbians' and gay men's mental health: Does sexual orientation really matter? *The American Psychologist, 56*(11), 931–947. doi:10.1037/0003-066X.56.11.931 PMID:11785169

Congress.gov. (2020). *H.R.5 – Equality Act, 116th Congress (2019–2020).* https://www.congress.gov/bill/116th-congress/house-bill/5

Drabble, L., & Trocki, K. (2005). Alcohol consumption, alcohol-related problems, and other substance use among lesbian and bisexual women. *Journal of Lesbian Studies, 9*(3), 19–30. doi:10.1300/J155v09n03_03 PMID:17548282

Federal Bureau of Investigation. (2018). *2018 hate crime statistics.* https://ucr.fbi.gov/hate-crime/2018/topic-pages/victims

Federal Safety Net. (2019). *U.S. poverty statistics-race.* http://federalsafetynet.com/us-poverty-statistics.html

Filmer, D. (2008). Disability, poverty, and schooling in developing countries: Results from 14 household surveys. *The World Bank Economic Review, 22*(1), 141–163. doi:10.1093/wber/lhm021

Glasper, A. (2016). Ensuring optimal health care for LGBT patients. *British Journal of Nursing (Mark Allen Publishing)*, *25*(13), 768–769. doi:10.12968/bjon.2016.25.13.768 PMID:27409790

Gruskin, E. P., & Gordon, N. (2006). Gay/Lesbian sexual orientation increases risk for cigarette smoking and heavy drinking among members of a large northern California health plan. *Biomedical Central Public Health, 6*, 241. https://bmcpublichealth.biomedcentral.com/articles/10.1186/1471-2458-6-241

Hausmann, L. R. M., Hannon, M. J., Kresevic, D. M., Hanusa, B. H., Kwoh, C. K., & Ibrahim, S. A. (2011). Impact of perceived discrimination in health care on patient–provider. *Communication. Medical Care*, *49*(7), 626–633. doi:10.1097/MLR.0b013e318215d93c PMID:21478769

Hendricks, M. L., & Testa, R. J. (2012). A conceptual framework for clinical work with transgender and gender nonconforming clients: An adaptation of the minority stress model. *Professional Psychology, Research and Practice*, *43*(5), 460–467. doi:10.1037/a0029597

Hiestand, K. R., Horne, S. G., & Levitt, H. M. (2007). Effects of gender identity on experiences of healthcare for sexual minority women. *Journal of LGBT Health Research*, *3*(4), 15–27. doi:10.1080/15574090802263405 PMID:19042908

Hoffman, K. M., Trawalter, S., Axt, J. R., & Oliver, M. N. (2016). Racial bias in pain assessment and treatment recommendations, and false beliefs about biological differences between Blacks and Whites. *Proceedings of the National Academy of Sciences of the United States of America*, *113*(16), 4296–4301. doi:10.1073/pnas.1516047113 PMID:27044069

Hommes, R. E., Borash, A. I., Hartwig, K., & DeGarcia, D. (2018). American Sign Language interpreters' perceptions of barriers to healthcare communication in deaf and hard of hearing patients. *Journal of Community Health*, *43*(5), 956–961. doi:10.100710900-018-0511-3 PMID:29696596

Howell, E. A. (2018). Reducing disparities in severe maternal morbidity and mortality. *Clinical Obstetrics and Gynecology*, *61*(2), 387–399. doi:10.1097/GRF.0000000000000349 PMID:29346121

Human Rights Campaign. (2021). *The Equality Act.* https://www.hrc.org/resources/the-equality-act

J. (2020). Talking about unconscious bias. *Kai Tiaki Nursing New Zealand, 26*(10), 32–33. https://issuu.com/kaitiaki/docs/kai_tiaki_november_2020

Jarlenski, M., Baller, J., Borrero, S., & Bennett, W. L. (2016). Trends in disparities in low-income children's health insurance coverage and access to care by family immigration status. *Academic Pediatrics, 16*(2), 208–215. doi:10.1016/j.acap.2015.07.008 PMID:26329016

Johnson, M. J., & Nemeth, L. S. (2014). Addressing health disparities of lesbian and bisexual women: A grounded theory study. *Women's Health Issues, 24*(6), 635–640. doi:10.1016/j.whi.2014.08.003 PMID:25287354

Kroenke, K., Spitzer, R. L., & Williams, J. W. (2001). The PHQ-9: Validity of a brief depression severity measure. *Journal of General Internal Medicine, 16*(9), 606–613. doi:10.1046/j.1525-1497.2001.016009606.x PMID:11556941

Lee, P., Le Saux, M., Siegel, R., Goyal, M., Chen, C., Ma, Y., & Meltzer, A. C. (2019). Racial and ethnic disparities in the management of acute pain in U.S. emergency departments: Meta-analysis and systematic review. *The American Journal of Emergency Medicine, 37*(9), 1770–1777. doi:10.1016/j.ajem.2019.06.014 PMID:31186154

Lefevor, G. T., Boyd-Rogers, C. C., & Janis, R. A. (2019). Health disparities between genderqueer, transgender, and cisgender individuals: An extension of minority stress theory. *Journal of Counseling Psychology, 66*(4), 385–395. doi:10.1037/cou0000339 PMID:30896208

Lowe, S. R., Tineo, P., & Young, M. N. (2018). Perceived discrimination and major depression and generalized anxiety symptoms in Muslim American college students. *Journal of Religion and Health, 58*(4), 1136–1145. doi:10.100710943-018-0684-1 PMID:30094677

Mahzarin, R., Banaji, A., & Greenwald, G. (2013). *Blindspot: Hidden biases of good people*. DelacortePress.

McEwen, B. (2005). Stressed or stressed out: What is the difference? *Journal of Psychiatry & Neuroscience, 30*(5), 315–318. doi:10.1055-0038-1675618 PMID:16151535

Meyer, I. H. (2003). Prejudice, social stress, and mental health in lesbian, gay, and bisexual populations: Conceptual issues and research evidence. *Psychological Bulletin, 129*(5), 674–697. doi:10.1037/0033-2909.129.5.674 PMID:12956539

Mizunoya, S., & Mitra, S. (2013). Is there a disability gap in employment rates in developing countries? *World Development*, *42*, 28–43. doi:10.1016/j.worlddev.2012.05.037

Mosack, K. E., Brouwer, A. M., & Petroll, A. E. (2013). Sexual identity, identity disclosure, and health care experience: Is there evidence for differential homophobia in primary care practice. *Women's Health Issues*, *23*(6), e341–e346. doi:10.1016/j.whi.2013.07.004 PMID:24183408

National Alliance to End Homelessness. (2020a). *State of homelessness 2020 edition*. https://endhomelessness.org/homelessness-in-america/homelessness-statistics/state-of-homelessness-2020/

National Alliance to End Homelessness. (2020b). *State of homelessness 2015 edition*. https://endhomelessness.org/the-state-of-homelessness-in-america-2015-trends-in-chronic-homelessness/

National Center for Health Statistics. (2017). *National Survey of Children's Health*. https://www.cdc.gov/nchs/slaits/nsch.htm

National Institute on Drug Abuse. (2020). *Opioid overdose crisis*. https://www.drugabuse.gov/drug-topics/opioids/opioid-overdose-crisis#:~:text=2018%20data%20shows%20that%20every,die%20after%20overdosing%20on%20opioids.&text=The%20misuse%20of%20and%20addiction,as%20social%20and%20economic%20welfare

National Institutes of Health, National Diabetes Program. (2006). *Silent trauma: Diabetes, health status, and the refugee: Southeast Asians in the United States*. https://ndep.nih.gov/media/SilentTrauma.pdf

Office of Disease Prevention and Health Promotion. (2020). *HealthyPeople.gov: Lesbian, gay, bisexual, and transgender health*. https://www.healthypeople.gov/2020/topics-objectives/topic/lesbian-gay-bisexual-and-transgender-health

Patriksson, K., Nilsson, S., & Wigert, H. (2019). Conditions for communication between health care professionals and parents on a neonatal ward in the presence of language barriers. *International Journal of Qualitative Studies on Health and Well-being*, *14*(1), 1–10. doi:10.1080/17482631.2019.1652060 PMID:31397216

Peled, Y. (2016). Language barriers and epistemic injustice in healthcare settings. *Bioethics*, *32*(6), 360–367. doi:10.1111/bioe.12435 PMID:29741210

Pew Research. (2019). *The countries with the 10 largest Christian populations and 10 largest Muslim populations*. Pew Research. https://www.pewresearch.org/fact-tank/2019/04/01/the-countries-with-the-10-largest-christian-populations-and-the-10-largest-muslim-populations/

Rogers, V. L., & Nesbitt, S. D. (2020). Overcoming racism and unconscious bias in OB/GYN practice. *Contemporary OB/GYN Journal, 64*(8), 15–17. https://www.contemporaryobgyn.net/view/overcoming-racism-and-unconscious-bias-in-ob-gyn

Shalowitz, M. U., Schetter, C. D., Hillemeier, M. M., Chinchilli, V. M., Adam, E. K., Hobel, C. J., Ramey, S. L., Vance, M. R., O'Campo, P., Thorp, J. M. Jr, Seeman, T. E., & Raju, T. N. K. (2019). Cardiovascular and metabolic risk in women in the first year postpartum: Allostatic load as a function of race, ethnicity, and poverty status. *American Journal of Perinatology, 36*(10), 1079–1089. doi:10.1055-0038-1675618 PMID:30551234

Showstack, R. (2019). Patients don't have language barriers; the healthcare system does. *Emergency Medicine Journal, 36*(10), 580–581. doi:10.1136/emermed-2019-208929 PMID:31405992

Sirin, S. R., & Fine, M. (2008). *Muslim American youth: Understanding hyphenated identities through multiple methods*. New York University Press.

Small, M. J., Allen, T. K., & Brown, H. L. (2017). Global disparities in maternal morbidity and mortality. *Seminars in Perinatology, 41*(5), 318–322. doi:10.1053/j.semperi.2017.04.009 PMID:28669415

Spitzer, R. L., Kroenke, K., Williams, J. W., & Lowe, B. (2006). A brief measure for assessing generalized anxiety disorder: The GAD-7. *Archives of Internal Medicine, 166*(10), 1092–1097. doi:10.1001/archinte.166.10.1092 PMID:16717171

Stevens, G. W. J. M., & Thijis, J. (2018). Perceived group discrimination and psychological well-being in ethnic minority adolescents. *Journal of Applied Social Psychology, 48*(10), 559–570. doi:10.1111/jasp.12547

Substance Abuse and Mental Health Services Administration. (2019). *2018 National Survey on Drug Use and Health: Methodological summary and definitions*. Center for Behavioral Health Statistics and Quality. https://www.samhsa.gov/data/sites/default/files/cbhsq-reports/NSDUHDetailedTabs2018R2/NSDUHDetailedTabs2018.pdf

Substance Abuse and Mental Health Services Administration. (2019). *2018 NSDUH detailed tables: National Survey on Drug Use and Health.* https://www.samhsa.gov/data/report/2018-nsduh-detailed-tables

Tempkin, S. M., Rimel, B. J., Bruegl, A. S., Gunderson, C. C., Beavis, A. L., & Doll, K. M. (2018). A contemporary framework of health equity applied to gynecologic cancer care: A Society of Gynecologic Oncology evidenced-based review. *Gynecologic Oncology, 149*(1), 70–77. doi:10.1016/j.ygyno.2017.11.013 PMID:29605053

The Patient Protection and Affordable Care Act, Publ. L. No. 111-148, 124 Stat. 119 (2010). https://www.govinfo.gov/content/pkg/PLAW-111publ148/pdf/PLAW-111publ148.pdf

United States Census. (2020). *2020 Census: LBTQ+.* https://www.census.gov/newsroom/press-kits/2020/2020-census-lgbtq.html

United States Department of Health and Human Services, Office of Minority Health. (2019a). *Mental and behavioral health – American Indians/Alaska Natives.* https://minorityhealth.hhs.gov/omh/browse.aspx?lvl=4&lvlid=39#2

United States Department of Health and Human Services, Office of Minority Health. (2019b). *Mental and behavioral health-Asian Americans.* https://minorityhealth.hhs.gov/omh/browse.aspx?lvl=4&lvlid=54#2

United States Department of Health and Human Services, Office of Minority Health. (2019c). *Mental health and behavioral health-African Americans.* https://www.minorityhealth.hhs.gov/omh/browse.aspx?lvl=4&lvlid=24

Ware, J. Jr, Kosinski, M., & Keller, S. D. (1996). A 12-item short-form health survey: Construction of scales and preliminary tests of reliability and validity. *Medical Care, 34*(3), 220–233. doi:10.1097/00005650-199603000-00003 PMID:8628042

Wilkerson, K., & Kirkwood, A. (2018). Unconscious bias: Getting rid of that pesky judgmental voice in your head. *Human Resources, 23*(1), 20–21.

Williams, D. R., Gonzalez, H. M., Williams, S., Mohammed, S. A., Moomal, H., & Stein, D. J. (2008). Perceived discrimination, race and health in South Africa. *Social Science & Medicine, 67*(3), 441–452. doi:10.1016/j.socscimed.2008.03.021 PMID:18486292

Chapter 5
Accessibility for All

ABSTRACT

Healthcare is a human necessity to maintain mental and physical health in modern society. Accessibility to healthcare is therefore a human right. However, it is a right that is not always granted or achievable. Not all Americans have insurance. The middle class and working poor must contend with high insurance premiums and out-of-pocket co-pays. Accessibility of healthcare information, symptom recognition, and disease management should be provided to at-risk populations, such as persons residing within rural or inner-city low-income areas, racial and ethnic minorities, and persons with literacy issues (i.e., unable to read or write). Lack of access to mental and physical healthcare can jeopardize individuals and, ultimately, the health and well-being of future generations.

LEARNING OBJECTIVES

1. Identify barriers associated with health care access.
2. Explain the importance of exploring the health care disparities of Arabic-speaking populations in the US.
3. Explain how Latinas experience discrimination while seeking sexual health care.
4. Discuss the importance of colorectal cancer screenings for immigrant workers and those that work off-hour shifts, making it difficult to access cancer screenings that are usually available during the daytime hours.

DOI: 10.4018/978-1-7998-3874-6.ch005

5. Differentiate the oral health care needs of persons diagnosed with human immunodeficiency virus (HIV) and acquired immunodeficiency syndrome (AIDS), older Americans, and veterans.
6. Discuss the importance of access to autism health care among transition-age youth.

Reflection Quote: "Access should not be a privilege for a few."

INTRODUCTION

Accessibility, when correlated with health care, speaks to persons having difficulty obtaining health services. Access can be impacted by poverty because the availability of monetary resources is limited, and affected persons are unable to purchase medications, medical equipment, health-care-related services, or transportation to attend health care appointments. For persons who have access issues, continuity with the management of diagnosed health care problems is complex and difficult. Labeled as **non-compliant** (refusal or failure to comply), persons who have difficulty paying for their health care needs must, at times, prioritize the purchasing of food or the payment of rent or a home mortgage over buying medication.

In discussing accessibility to health care, there are multiple factors that impact persons' ability to acquire health care services. Travel to the health facility, center, or office may be impeded by not having a car or being far from to public transportation. Clients may also be reliant on a livery medical cab or van paid by Medicaid for transportation to health care appointments. The **Medicaid non-emergency medical transport (NEMT)** is provided to Medicaid beneficiaries who require transportation to medical appointments. However, appointments must be scheduled in advance. With regard to medical emergencies, such as a stroke or heart attack, Medicaid will provide transportation by medical flight (air) or ambulance (ground) services (Center for Medicare and Medicaid Services, 2016). Insurance affordability, poverty, mental and physical disabilities, and lack of available and affordable health care services remain a problem in the US and abroad, impacting children and adults alike.

THE PATIENT PROTECTION AND AFFORDABLE CARE ACT

Kaye (2019) examined the impact of the **Patient Protection and Affordable Care Act (ACA)** on decreasing health disparities in the US since its inception in 2010. The aim of the ACA was to expand health insurance coverage to the public by improving the affordability of and access to private insurance. Provisions for uninsured persons included: (1) coverage of persons with pre-existing conditions at lower costs, with prohibitions against denial of coverage; (2) increasing Medicaid limits for low-income families and subsidizing the cost of private insurance; and (3) extending coverage to younger adults who are included in their parents' private insurance plans.

While the ACA was successful in helping many more people gain access to health care based on age, socioeconomic status (SES), and disability, disparities remain. Gaps in coverage remain, in particular, for persons with disabilities and risks for delays in care, mental illness disabilities, and persons/families who fall into income gaps created because Medicaid coverage is not consistent across states (Kaye, 2019). According to Kaye (2019), because racial and ethnic disparities remain a problem in the US, these disparities must also be addressed by policies to further improve the ACA.

BARRIERS TO HEALTH CARE ACCESS

Access to health care can be attributed to linguistic barriers, sex, gender, or identity stereotypes, and medical diagnoses that carry stigma in relation to the most statistically impacted impoverished or racial/ethnic minority groups. Be it oral health, sexual health, or cancer screenings, access must be prioritized to resolve health disparities. To improve access, we must first identify persons and health-related areas that are affected.

Access to Health Care in the US Territories

There are currently five major territories under the authority of the US that are partially self-governed. They are: Puerto Rico, Guam, the US Virgin Islands, America Samoa, and the Northern Mariana Islands. For these territories, their distance from the US affects access to quality health care. Higher mortality 30-day rates and poor performance on core process measures were observed in

US territories. Persons admitted with the diagnoses of heart failure, myocardial infarction, and pneumonia were more likely to die of complications. While some hospitals in Puerto Rico have the same performance achievements as state-side hospitals, for both Puerto Rico and the US Virgin Islands, gaps in care remain a problem. For example, in these territories there are low numbers of intensive care unit beds and fewer registered nurses and emergency medicine specialists (Hirshon et al., 2014; Rodriguez-Vila et al., 2017).

Stereotypes of Latinas Seeking Access to Sexual Health Care

Morales-Aleman et al. (2020) conducted community-based participatory research on how young Latinas experience sexual health care in Alabama. Semi-structured interviews with 20 Latinas aged 15–19 years who had resided in the US for five or more years were completed. The data were analyzed using the Socioecological Model of Sexual Health (SEMSH). Although 60% of the Latinas had health insurance and 65% were born in the US, the women reported embarrassment around inappropriate inquiries about their sexual health, stigmatization, and discrimination.

Health Care Barriers for Arabic-Speaking Populations

The Arabic language is used in the writing of the Koran, the religious text of Islam, and is a South-Central Semitic (Afro-Asiatic) language. The population of Arab Americans is growing. In 2017, there were an estimated 3.7 million Arab Americans in the US. However, health data on Arab Americans is not well documented because, like many minorities, there are no specific identifiers in electronic medical records or health surveys denoting this particular group as being Arab. Hence, health care data on illness and disease trends are limited (Al Jumaili et al., 2020).

Al Jumaili et al. (2020) conducted a cross-sectional study of native Arabic-speaking adults in Johnson County, Iowa. The purpose of the study was to assess health literacy, measure the prevalence of Arab Americans seeking preventive health services, and identify barriers to health care access. Two methods of data collection were used: an anonymous survey and a focus group that took place at a mosque in Iowa City.

The results indicated that, of the 196 participants, 52.6% reported having preventive health care visits with a physician, and 70% shared that they see a physician only when they are very ill. Forty-three percent stated that they encountered language barriers while seeking health care, had very high insurance co-pays, or had no insurance. Participants with health insurance (64.8%) were more likely to regularly visit their physicians, while those who did not have insurance (81.1%) did not regularly have physician visits or engage in preventive health care visits. In exploring chronic diseases, 32.7% of the participants had been diagnosed with one or more of the following: arthritis, asthma, hypertension, heart disease, and diabetes mellitus. The most common chronic disease diagnoses were diabetes mellitus (11.2%) and hypertension (15.3%) (Al Jumaili et al., 2020).

Access to Oral Healthcare by Persons with HIV/AIDS

Persons diagnosed with HIV or AIDS experience discrimination (Donnelly et al., 2016) surrounding fears of disease contagion and how the virus was contracted (i.e., from multiple sexual partners or intravenous drug use). Dental professionals, such as dentists, oral surgeons, and hygienists, working with individuals diagnosed with HIV/AIDS are required to take the same precautions as they would with all other patients to protect themselves from blood and body fluids. The source of the virus—for example, whether it was obtained through a blood transfusion during acute illness in a hospital setting, molestation, or during the birthing process—is irrelevant.

In 2016, it was estimated that 63,110 people residing in Canada had HIV (Public Health Agency of Canada, 2018; British Columbia Centre for Disease Control, 2017). Feng et al. (2019) examined data from a preventive oral health program that was developed by the University of British Columbia (UBC) Dental Hygiene Program in 2011 for the Positive Living Society of British Columbia (PLSBC). The purpose of the UBC and PLSBC collaboration was to improve access to oral health care for persons living with HIV/AIDS. Study participants included 12 staff and 10 PLSBC members. Feng et al. (2019) applied an interpretive phenomenology approach that followed access theory, which was developed by Penchansky and Thomas (1981).

The findings indicated that persons living with HIV, identified as members (n = 10), who had previously experienced trauma through stigmatization after indicating they were HIV-positive, reported feeling welcomed and accepted in the UBC/PLSBC program. The dental hygiene students, because of their education and interactions on the subject of cultural sensitivity about HIV, felt more comfortable caring for persons diagnosed with HIV/AIDS. The members participants who were either underemployed (i.e., part-time positions with minimum to no insurance) or unemployed could not afford dental care. Because the UBC and PLSBC oral hygiene care was free, members participants were able to save money for preventive oral care. Additionally, with regard to location of the oral hygiene program, it was located in Downtown Vancouver, and easily accessible through public transportation.

Access to Oral Health Care by Older Americans

Orozco et al. (2019) noted that oral health remains inaccessible to many low-income people over the age of 65 years. The National Health and Nutrition Examination Surveys between the years of 2009 and 2014 found that, in the US, approximately 18% of older Americans had lost all of their teeth (Dye et al., 2019). However, in 1957, data on oral health revealed that over 55% of older Americans had lost all of their teeth (Dye et al., 2019; Slade et al., 2014).

For older Americans with comorbidities, such as cardiovascular disease, diabetes mellitus, obesity, and malnutrition, the development of oral diseases, infections, and complications is higher (Jacobsen & Chavez, 2005; Teshome & Yitayeh, 2017). It is therefore imperative that oral health be included in state and federal policies related to preventive and primary health care. An example of oral health care focused on the older adult is the Gary and Mary West Senior Dental Center in San Diego, California. Over 500 older adults who do not have a provider that accepts Medicaid for dental care, or access to transportation, and are low income, receive oral health care at the center. The center is a model for oral health access that can be duplicated in other states in the US.

Access to Oral Health Care by Veterans

Suman et al. (2008) conducted a study on the impact of war on the oral health of soldiers. Study participants consisted of 640 soldiers in the Croatian Army; the control group included 304 peacetime soldiers, and the study group included 336 soldiers in active service (1991–1997). Participants were provided questionnaires about their oral health, including the Community Periodontal Index and the Decayed, Missing, and Filled Teeth Index, as well as diet and dental behaviors. The findings indicated that soldiers engaged in war were more likely to have poor oral health. Periodontal disease, poor diet, and a decreased frequency of teeth brushing were consistent issues with active-service soldiers. Overall, increased time in combat situations was correlated with poor oral health.

Oral healthcare is not accessible to all US veterans through the Veterans Affairs Dental Care program. Dental benefits are associated with service time provided by the individual veteran. A cross-sectional study was conducted by Nieto et al. (2019) with 227 veterans from Michigan using a 24-item survey. The surveys were provided in person to veterans over the course of two months. The survey inquired about information such as the ability to pay for dental care, the veteran's status of oral health (good or poor), and whether a toothache was present over the 12 months before study participation. With a participant response rate of 80% (n = 182), veterans who did not have an identified dentist (or place to receive dental care) or who could not afford dental care perceived themselves as having poor oral care and had a toothache in the last 12 months. These factors were identified as oral health disparities.

Colorectal Screenings and Access to Health Care

The current average age for colorectal cancer screening is 45 years (American Cancer Society, 2018). At this time, screenings include stool-based testing and colonoscopy. Costas-Muniz et al. (2019) examined how occupation, sociodemographic, health-related factors, and migration can impact the completion of colorectal screening. The authors studied 137 male taxi drivers in New York City and found that 27% had colorectal screenings completed. The findings revealed that the barriers to receiving colorectal screenings for the taxi drivers were driving high numbers of hours weekly and working night shifts. Taxi drivers, many of whom immigrated to the US, were more likely to obtain colorectal cancer screening if they had health insurance, a family history of cancer, had a routine health assessment (physical exam) in the last year, and had an identified regular source of primary care.

Access to Autism Health Care among Transition-Age Youth

In the US, 1 in 54 children has autism (CDC, 2020). The average age for identification of autism is eight years. Signs and symptoms of autism are more than four times as likely to be identified in boys than girls, but girls diagnosed with autism tend to have more intellectual disabilities (32% of boys; 39% of girls) than their male counterparts. Autism impacts persons of all SES levels, races, and ethnicities. While racial gaps in diagnoses among Latinx and Black children have gradually closed, the former are diagnosed at lower rates than the latter. Of concern is that late diagnoses still occur with non-White children. White children are more likely to receive an early diagnosis and, hence, early treatment with better outcomes than Black or Latinx children (CDC, 2020).

Iannuzzi et al. (2018) used a mixed-methods randomized controlled trial pilot study to evaluate an educational curriculum developed to address the medical needs of transition-age youth (TAY) diagnosed with autism. Participants in the study were 14 family nurse practitioner students who were assigned randomly to an intervention group (INT, n = 6) or a waitlist control group (WLC, n = 8). Qualitative and quantitative data were gathered. Attitude (3.1 INT and −6.25 WLC, mean standard deviations), knowledge (7.91 INT and −3.43 WLC, mean standard deviations), and self-efficacy (42.7 INT and 5.19 WLC, mean standard deviations) measurements were used for the pre- and posttests. The Qualitative and Quantitative data were gathered. Study findings indicated that the family nurse practitioner students positively benefited from the educational curriculum developed on TAY diagnosed with autism; as a result, the curriculum was adopted into the nurse practitioner, family nurse practitioner, and adult-gerontology primary care nurse practitioner programs at the University of Massachusetts.

When children and youths with autism no longer are of age to continue receiving medical care from a pediatrician, transitioning to an adult primary care provider can be difficult because not all adult health care providers are trained in the care of persons with autism. Autism and other developmental disorders are content areas that require additional training and ongoing educational support to prepare adult health care providers to care for the complex behavioral, physical, and emotional changes experienced by persons diagnosed with autism (Bruder et al., 2012; Iannuzzi et al., 2019; Patel & O'Hare, 2010). TAYs with autism may have seizures, intellectual disabilities, sensory-processing issues, sleep disorders, gastrointestinal disorders, and be hypersensitive to tactile, auditory, and visual stimuli (Aylott, 2010; Bauman, 2010; Buie et al., 2010). Hence, education on autism is needed by adult health providers to meet the health care needs of youth transitioning to adult health care services.

SUMMARY

Access to health care systems can be obstructed by lack of client knowledge of health care information, finances, no insurance or being underinsured, lack of knowledge by health care providers, transportation, language barriers, racism, stereotyping, and discrimination. Access infers entering freely and without complication. However, access in health care is a fallacy if selected groups of people are granted health care in absence of obstacles, while others are not.

Figure 1. Obstacles to access

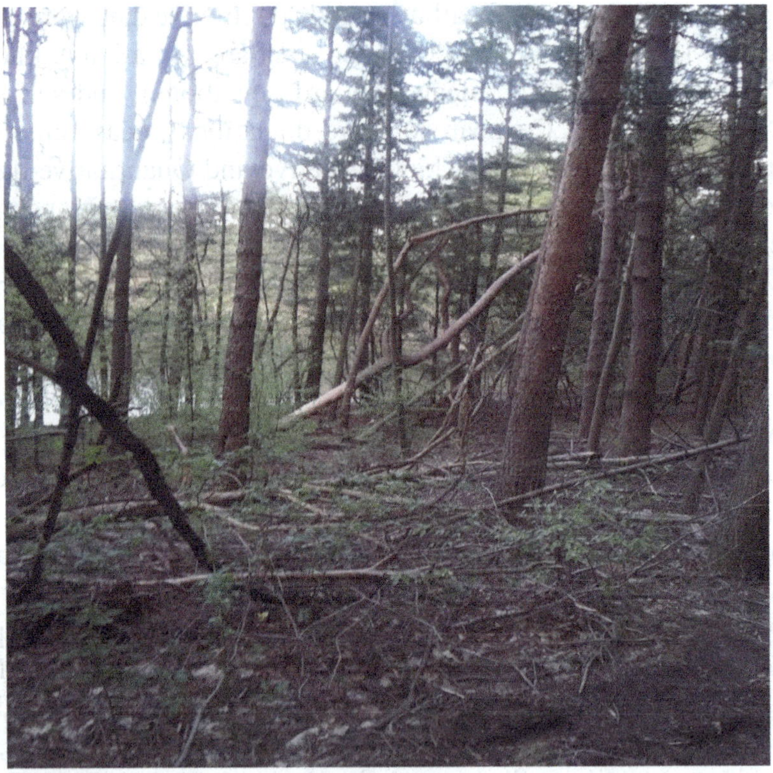

ACCESS TO HEALTHCARE

Directions: Review the questions and statements below. Determine why health care access remains a problem for so many people in the US. Consider what can be implemented to change this occurrence at a systems level in organizations, towns, cities, and rural areas. Is access a federal issue, or should resolution originate from local and state governments?

1. Is health care access an achievable goal for all Americans?
2. Veterans serve the citizens of the US. Should access for all veterans be resolved at the organizational systems level through cooperative agreements with the federal government, military, and the Veterans Affairs medical centers?
3. How do racism and discrimination affect health care access?
4. Why are language barriers still a health care access issue when health care facilities have electronic technologies, telephone systems, and in-person translators to facilitate communication?
5. Should health care providers be held accountable for lack of knowledge regarding clients' diagnoses that affect their ability to provide evidenced-based health care?
6. How do stereotypes impact clients' access to health care?
7. What mechanisms are in place in most healthcare systems for clients to report difficulties in accessing health care?
8. How does lack of finances and insurance impact individuals' and families' access to health care?
9. How can the US improve access to health care resources, like registered nurses and emergency care specialists, for the five US territories?
10. Should the five US territories seek ways to draw qualified health care professionals and health care organizations and facilities to their island locations to improve access for their residents?

CASE STUDY: ACCESS TO COLORECTAL SCREENING

I finally got insurance through my job and I need to get screened for colon cancer. My father died of this type of cancer at 45 years of age, and I am 42 years old. My problem is that I work night and evening shifts as a cab driver and sleep during the day. I try to schedule appointments for my day off, but there are very few available. What can I do but wait several months to finally get my cancer screening done?

Discussion: *Should insured Americans who pay an insurance premium to companies to receive preventive healthcare services have access to more frequent and off-hour medical screenings?*

Figure 2. Access barriers

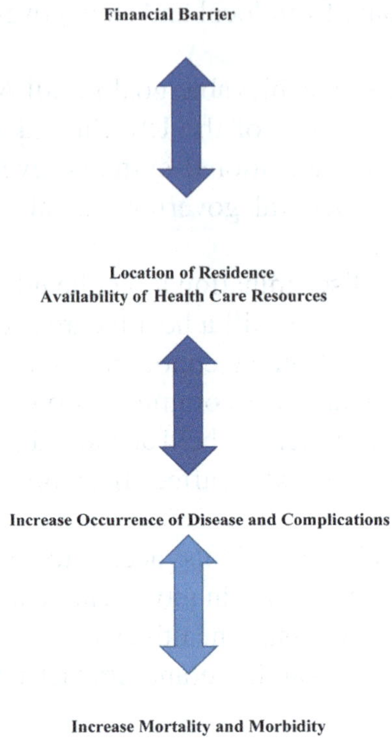

REFERENCES

Al Jumaili, A. A., Ahmed, K. K., & Koch, D. (2020). Barriers to healthcare access for Arabic-speaking populations in an English-speaking country. *Pharmacy Practice*, *18*(2), 1–8. doi:10.18549/PharmPract.2020.2.1809 PMID:32477432

American Cancer Society. (2018). *American Cancer Society updates colorectal screening guideline*. https://www.cancer.org/latest-news/american-cancer-society-updates-colorectal-cancer-screening-guideline.html#:~:text=The%20American%20Cancer%20Society%20%28ACS%29%20has%20released%20an,at%20age%2050%20for%20people%20at%20average%20risk

Aylott, J. (2010). Improving access to health and social care for people with autism. *Nursing Standard*, *24*(27), 47–56. doi:10.7748/ns.24.27.47.s57 PMID:20373630

Bauman, M. L. (2010). Medical comorbidities in autism: Challenges to diagnosis and treatment. *Neurotherapeutics; the Journal of the American Society for Experimental NeuroTherapeutics*, *7*(3), 320–327. doi:10.1016/j.nurt.2010.06.001 PMID:20643385

British Columbia Centre for Disease Control. (2017). *HIV in British Columbia: Annual surveillance report 2016*. http://www.bccdc.ca/resource-gallery/Documents/Statistics%20and%20Research/Statistics%20and%20Reports/STI/HIV_Annual_Report_2016.pdf

Bruder, M. B., Kerins, G., Mazzarella, C., Sims, J., & Stein, N. (2012). Brief report: The medical care of adults with autism spectrum disorders: Identifying the needs. *Journal of Autism and Developmental Disorders*, *42*(11), 2498–2504. doi:10.100710803-012-1496-x PMID:22427260

Buie, T., Campbell, D., Fuchs, G. III, Furuta, G., Levy, J., VandeWater, J., Whitaker, A. H., Atkins, D., Bauman, M. L., Beaudet, A. L., Carr, E. G., Gershon, M. D., Hyman, S. L., Jirapinyo, P., Jyonouchi, H., Kooros, K., Kushak, R., Levitt, P., Levy, S. E., ... Winter, H. (2010). Evaluation, diagnosis and treatment of gastrointestinal disorders in individuals with ASDs: A consensus report. *Pediatrics*, *125*(Suppl 1), S1–S18. doi:10.1542/peds.2009-1878C PMID:20048083

Centers for Disease Control and Prevention. (2020). *Autism prevalence rises in communities monitored by the CDC*. https://www.cdc.gov/media/releases/2020/p0326-autism-prevalence-rises.html

Centers for Medicare and Medicaid Services. (2016). *Fact sheet: Let Medicaid give you a ride*. https://www.cms.gov/Medicare-Medicaid-Coordination/Fraud-Prevention/Medicaid-Integrity-Education/Downloads/nemt-factsheet.pdf

Costas-Muniz, R., Roberts, N., Narang, B., Mehmood, R., Acharya, S., Aragones, A., Leng, J., & Gany, F. (2019). Colorectal cancer screening and access to healthcare in New York City taxi drivers. *Journal of Immigrant and Minority Health*, *22*(3), 526–533. doi:10.100710903-019-00911-8 PMID:31263989

Donnelly, L. R., Bailey, L., Jessani, A., Postnikoff, J., Kerston, P., & Brondani, M. (2016). Stigma experiences in marginalized people living with HIV seeking health services and resources in Canada. *The Journal of the Association of Nurses in AIDS Care: JANAC, 26*(6), 768–783. doi:10.1016/j.jana.2016.07.003 PMID:27554334

Dye, B. A., Weatherspoon, D. J., & Mitnik, G. L. (2019). Tooth loss among older adults according to poverty status in the United States from 1999 through 2004 and 2009 through 2014. *The Journal of the American Dental Association, 150*(1), 9–23. doi:10.1016/j.adaj.2018.09.010 PMID:30503018

Feng, I., Brondani, M., Bedos, C., & Donnelly, L. (2019). Access to oral health care for people living with HIV/AIDS attending a community-based program. *Canadian Journal of Dental Hygiene, 54*(1), 7–15. PMID:33240359

Hirshon, J. M., Alson, R. L., Blunk, D., Brosnan, D. P., Epstein, S. K., Gardner, A. F., Lum, D. L., Moskovitz, J. B., Richardson, L. D., Stankus, J. L., & Kivela, P. D. (n.d.). *America's emergency care environment: A state-by-state report card.* http://www.emreportcard.org/uploadedFiles/EMReportCard2014.pdf

Iannuzzi, D. A., Cheng, E. R., Broder-Fingert, S., & Bauman, M. L. (2014). Brief report: Emergency department utilization by individuals with autism. *Journal of Autism and Developmental Disorders, 45*(4), 1096–1102. doi:10.100710803-014-2251-2 PMID:25261249

Iannuzzi, D. A., Rissmiller, P., Duty, S. M., Feeney, S., Sullivan, M., & Curtin, C. (2019). Addressing a gap in healthcare access for transition-age youth with autism: A pilot educational intervention for family nurse practitioner students. *Journal of Autism and Developmental Disorders, 49*(4), 1493–1504. doi:10.100710803-018-3846-9 PMID:30536218

Jacobsen, P. L., & Chavez, E. M. (2005). Clinical management of the dental patient taking multiple drugs. *The Journal of Contemporary Dental Practice, 6*(4), 144–151. doi:10.5005/jcdp-6-4-144 PMID:16299616

Kaye, S. (2019). Disability-related disparities in access to health care before (2008–2010) and after (2015–2017) the Affordable Care Act. *American Journal of Public Health, 109*(7), 1015–1021. doi:10.2105/AJPH.2019.305056 PMID:31095413

Morales-Aleman, M. M., Ferreti, G., & Scaricini, I. C. (2020). "I don't like being stereotyped, I decided I was going back to the doctor": Sexual healthcare access among young Latina women in Alabama. *Journal of Immigrant and Minority Health, 22*(4), 645–652. doi:10.100710903-019-00932-3 PMID:31535273

National Institutes of Health. (2021). *Cultural respect.* https://www.nih.gov/institutes-nih/nih-office-director/office-communications-public-liaison/clear-communication/cultural- respect#:~:text=Culture%20is%20often%20described%20as,%2C%20geographic%2C%20or%20social%20groups

Nieto, V., Arnett, M., & Furgeson, D. (2019). Attitudes and access patterns of Michigan veterans ineligible for oral healthcare benefits: A cross-sectional study. *American Dental Hygienists Association, 93*(4), 6–13. PMID:31409719

Orozco, M., Becerra, K., & Shumulinsky, V. (2019). Improving access to oral healthcare among low-income older adults. *Generations: Journal of the American Society on Aging*, 70–74. https://www.pcpcc.org/sites/default/files/resources/Oral%20Health%20in%20Older%20Adults.pdf

Patel, M. S., & O'Hare, K. (2010). Residency training in transition of youth with childhood-onset chronic disease. *Pediatrics, 126*(Suppl 3), S190–S193. doi:10.1542/peds.2010-1466P PMID:21123485

Penchansky, R., & Thomas, J. W. (1981). The concept of access: Definition and relationship to Consumer satisfaction. *Medical Care, 19*(2), 127–140. doi:10.1097/00005650-198102000-00001 PMID:7206846

Public Health Agency of Canada. (2018). *Estimates of HIV incidence, prevalence and Canada's progress on meeting the 90-90-90 HIV targets, 2016.* https://www.canada.ca/en/services/health/publications/diseases-conditions/hiv-surveillance-infographic-2017.html

Rodriquez-Vila, O., Nuti, S. V., & Keomkolz, H. M. (2017). Health disparities affecting Americans in the U.S. territories: A century-old dilemma. *The American Journal of Medicine, 130*(2), E39–E42. doi:10.1016/j.amjmed.2016.07.036 PMID:27593609

Slade, G., Akinkugbe, A., & Sanders, A. (2014). Projections of U.S. edentulism prevalence following five decades of decline. *Journal of Dental Research, 93*(10), 958–965. doi:10.1177/0022034514546165 PMID:25146182

Suman, M., Spalj, S., Plancak, D., Dukic, W., & Juric, H. (2008). The influence of war on the health of professional soldiers. *International Dental Journal*, *58*(2), 71–74. doi:10.1111/j.1875-595X.2008.tb00178.x PMID:18478886

Teshome, A., & Yiyateh, A. (2017). The effect of periodontal therapy on glycemic control and fasting plasma glucose level in type 2 diabetic patients: Systematic review and meta-analysis. *BMC Oral Health*, *17*(1), 31. doi:10.118612903-016-0249-1 PMID:27473177

Chapter 6
A Solution

ABSTRACT

The solutions to end health disparities are complex and involve introspection and confrontation with one's own perceived beliefs about our fellow human beings who are of a different socioeconomic status, sex, religion, age, gender, and physical appearance than ourselves. No person, even if of the same skin color and culture, is the same. Hence, the solution to health disparities is the societal decision to hold accountable those who harm others by withholding health information and treatment that can sustain and prolong life. The value of all human lives is priceless. Hence, access to healthcare and quality evidenced-based care is a right for all.

LEARNING OBJECTIVES

1. Discuss the importance of recognizing the human species as one of solidarity.
2. Explain why states and the federal government should work collaboratively as gatekeepers in holding health care organizations, workers, and providers accountable for high numbers of health disparity issues arising within their facilities.
3. Explore ways in which health care consumers can participate in ensuring that they are in fact receiving quality, evidenced-based health care.

DOI: 10.4018/978-1-7998-3874-6.ch006

Reflection Quote: "I told my doctor, if I had a car I could make all my appointments. Trying to walk to the bus stop with a quad cane and a limp can be a little difficult. The livery cab is not always available when I need to use it on short notice."

INTRODUCTION

A human being is a member of the species ***Homo sapiens***. Lattal (2017), in posing the concept of **human-as-instrument**, examines *H. sapiens* using a scientific instrument that has the ability to measure the behavioral aspects of punishment and contingencies of reinforcement. Because *H. sapiens* are social beings (Harris, 2005) who prefer to congregate and communicate in groups, the acceptance of one another based upon group similarities or common interests often prevails.

Instinctual Social Acceptance

Theoretically, *H. sapiens's* tendency to congregate socially with others who are similar, lends itself to the historical problems of racism and discrimination. However, it is ironic that *H. sapiens* represents a species of human beings, which includes everyone. In theory, then, group members should not consider differences in their peers as the biological rationale for racism and discrimination, lest they discriminate against their very existence.

Foundations for Change

Health disparities have a long history in the US. Chapter 2 explored the unethical experiments performed on humans by researchers and how these studies compromised the patients' health and safety. The experiments include those performed on Jews imprisoned in concentration camps by the Nazis. Jews, members of the species *H. sapiens*, had drugs tested on them; were given poisons, malaria, and typhus; were sterilized, exposed to freezing temperatures and high altitudes; and euthanized. Treated inhumanely by their captors, Jews were given surgeries that were neither medically nor surgically indicated and performed without anesthesia (Berger, 1990; Steinfels & Levine, 1976; Weindling, 2005).

African American men, also members of *H. sapiens*, were seen by physicians who withheld treatment for syphilis, a bacterial sexually transmitted infection, during the US Public Health Service Tuskegee Syphilis Study in 1932. Left untreated, syphilis causes multiple long-term complications, including stroke, psychosis, meningitis, paresis (as a result of aortitis, inflammation of the aortic wall), neurosyphilis, and dementia (Grossman & Porth, 2014; Hinkle & Cheever 2018; Rothman, 1982)

In Staten Island, New York, during the mid-1950s through the early 1970s, children and adults with disabilities, members of *H. sapiens*, were intentionally exposed to the hepatitis virus during an unethical study at the Willowbrook State Developmental Center (Disability Justice, 2020; Rothman, 1982). Likewise, a study conducted in 1962 at the Jewish Chronic Disease Hospital in Brooklyn, New York, explored the immune response of patients, also *H. sapiens*, who were diagnosed with cancer to the injection of live cancer cells into their bodies (Hershey & Miller, 1976; Levine, 1986; Alliance for Research Protection, 2020).

Moving Forward Toward a Solution

Our historical foundations for social change in the US have been formed by the injustices experienced by *H. sapiens* at the hands of their peers. Though the species is united biologically, our different characteristics are often used to separate, confine, and despise others based on genetic variations in physical presentation that are affected by geographical location; genetics and genomics.

Regulations and laws have been formulated over the years to protect research subjects from unethical experimentation (Beecher, 1966; Brandt, 1978; Berger, 1990). This is why Institutional Review Boards (IRBs) exist in academia and organizations to protect the rights of research participants (Constantin, 2018). However, health disparities persist and have been identified by the US government (ODPHP, 2020) among vulnerable populations, such as children, the elderly, the un- and underinsured, persons with certain medical conditions, socioeconomically disadvantaged people, and racial and ethnic minorities (Waisel, 2013). Historically, members of these groups have been the recipients of poor health care. Unfortunately, health equity remains an issue because not all Americans are guaranteed quality care. The solution lies in our data identifying at-risk and vulnerable populations. These very data highlight our weaknesses as a country with significant health disparities, but they can be used to decrease these disparities in each state.

The US Department of Health and Human Services (DHHS) oversees the Centers for Medicare and Medicaid Services (CMS). In 2017, spending for the Medicare program totaled $705.9 billion and covered over 58 million people (Medicare.gov, 2020a). Monies for the Medicare program are managed by the US Treasury and consist of two trust funds: the **hospital insurance trust fund** and the **supplementary medical insurance trust fund**. The hospital insurance trust fund monies originate from income taxes paid on social security benefits, Medicare Part A premiums (hospital insurance) for persons who do not qualify for premium-free Part A, payroll taxes, and interest earned on trust fund investments. Supplementary medical insurance trust fund monies originate from interest earned on trust fund investments, funds authorized by Congress, and the premiums from persons enrolled in Medicare Part B (medical insurance) and Medicare prescription drug coverage (Part D; Medicare.gov, 2020a).

The states and federal government, together, fund the Medicaid health program, with the federal government paying the Federal Medical Assistance Percentage, or the percentage of monies paid based on services and care delivered. Currently, states are permitted to determine the amounts that Medicaid health care providers receive, as long as the rates of provider payments fall within guidelines set by the federal government (Medicaid.gov, 2020a). Each month, the 50 states (and the District of Columbia) are required to provide enrollment activity and eligibility data on the Children's Health Insurance Program (CHIP) and Medicaid. For example, in March of 2020, nationally, there were 70,887,950 persons enrolled in the CHIP and Medicaid programs; 6,793,209 were enrolled in CHIP, and 64,094,741 were enrolled in Medicaid (Medicaid.gov, 2020b).

Health disparities and inequities can be resolved at the state level if determinants for success and evidence of equitable services rendered are directly correlated with states receiving Medicare and Medicaid funding for health care services provided within each state. When there are significant variations in health services rendered to vulnerable populations across regions within a state, the state is required to investigate the origins of these disparities within three months. Upon completion of the investigation, if health disparities remain unchanged over the course of 6–12 months, the state must hold health care organizations accountable by issuing a fine.

It is by holding individual states accountable for health disparities through the penalty of fines that health care inequities can be addressed. With regard to the federal government's involvement, by placing a weighted percentage based on those identified in the Healthy People Initiative (ODPHP, 2020), the prevalence of health disparities throughout the US can be quantified and, at the state level, brought to fruition by monthly data monitoring. Such monitoring would be in line with the existing monthly data gathered through the CHIP and Medicaid programs for eligibility and enrollment. For the Medicare program, monthly data review would expedite payment for services rendered and identify substandard treatment potentially impacting morbidity and mortality in vulnerable populations.

EDUCATING HEALTH CARE WORKERS AND PROVIDERS FOR CHANGE

Holding health care workers and providers accountable for awareness, knowledge, and application to clinical practice of health disparities must be an essential part of the training of nurses, physicians, physician assistants, nurse assistants, respiratory therapists, physical therapists, psychologists, social workers, podiatrists, psychiatrists, occupational therapists, dieticians, optometrists, physiatrists, dentists, and all other healthcare professionals. Hence, educational institutions offering coursework in health care specialties must demonstrate evidence of such training to receive funding from the federal government. Specifically, evidence must show the offering of courses and coursework addressing health disparities, discrimination in health care against vulnerable populations, and identification of risk factors contributing to chronic disease among racial and ethnic minorities and persons of low SES. When professionals understand risk factors, such as age, sex, obesity, tobacco use, sedentary lifestyle, alcohol use, chronic stress, occupational hazards, nutrition, and environmental and chemical exposures in vulnerable populations, chronic disease (e.g., diabetes mellitus, asthma, stroke, Alzheimer's disease, cancer, chronic obstructive pulmonary disease, chronic kidney disease, and heart disease) can be prevented (CDC, 2019).

Health promotion and prevention of disease must be at the forefront of all health care workers' and providers' educational training to decrease or eliminate health care disparities. The annual cost of health care in the US is approximately \$3.5 trillion, with chronic diseases being the leading cause of disability and deaths. Ninety percent of the \$3.5 trillion is attributed to chronic health and mental health conditions (CDC, 2020; National Center for Chronic Disease and Health Promotion, 2020).

In examining the costs incurred by the US for chronic diseases, the following data for 2020 were noted: 88 million Americans have pre-diabetes that could lead to type 2 diabetes, and 34.2 million have diabetes mellitus; the total cost incurred by the nation in 2017 for diabetes mellitus in terms of lost productivity and medical costs was \$327 billion. Cancer care costs are rising and were estimated at \$174 billion in 2020, with 600,000 people dying from cancer and 1.6 million people being newly diagnosed. Epilepsy affects 470,000 teenagers and children and 3 million adults; annually, the cost per affected person ranges from \$10,200 to \$47,900 (2013 data). Stroke and heart disease cost Americans \$131 billion each year in productive time on the job; they kill 859,000 people annually and cost the healthcare system \$199 billion for stroke and heart disease care. Approximately \$304 billion was spent in 2013 on arthritis care; \$164 billion was the result of lost earnings, and \$140 billion went to medical costs. At this time, 54.4 million adults are affected by arthritis in the US (National Center for Chronic Disease and Health Promotion, 2020).

The annual cost for the problem of obesity in the US is \$147 billion. Obesity places adults and children at risk for chronic diseases. Lack of physical activity contributes to the development of obesity, cancers, heart disease, and type 2 diabetes. The cost associated with lack of physical activity annually is \$117 billion. Over 60 million people in the US have a disease associated with smoking, with \$170 billion in medical costs. The US economy was estimated to be negatively impacted in 2010 by alcohol abuse, totaling \$249 billion, with 88,000 Americans dying annually from alcohol-related deaths (National Center for Chronic Disease and Health Promotion, 2020).

In older Americans, **Alzheimer's disease**, a progressive dementia, affects approximately 5.7 million people. Estimates for treatment of adults diagnosed with Alzheimer's disease were between \$159 billion and \$215 billion. Alzheimer's disease costs are projected to increase by 2040 to between \$379 billion and \$500 billion each year. Tooth decay effects one in four adults and one in five children 11 years of age. Dental decay can impact learning, cause pain, and affect speaking and eating. For adults, over \$45 billion is lost in work productivity related to dental problems, and for children, approximately 34 million hours of school are lost each year as a result of the need for emergency dental care (National Center for Chronic Disease and Health Promotion, 2020).

Consumer Responsibility

Consumers of health care, once provided education on health disparities by their health providers, are accountable for their own health maintenance. Accountability includes formulating care plans to identify, explain, and reduce risk factors associated with chronic disease development. The care plans would be realistic in the measured time limits for the achievement of goals, and mutually agreed upon and signed by the health care provider and the consumer. Failure to achieve the goals over the period of three years could result in a scaled (increased) premium payment by consumers to their private health insurance companies, Medicare, and Medicaid. The scaled premium payments would be based on monthly income and determined by individual states.

SUMMARY

The solutions to health disparities lie in being accountable to the existing data that identify vulnerable populations as consumers of health care who must engage in rectifying their risk factors for chronic disease. Illness is not the sole responsibility of the providers of health care, or the insurance companies, but must engage all involved entities (i.e., individual consumers, private insurance companies, Medicaid, Medicare, the states, and the federal government). The longevity of health disparities in the US that cost trillions of dollars is illogical given that we have the science, treatments, and therapeutic interventions available to prevent chronic disease.

Health Disparity Solutions

Directions: As you read and answer each question, consider how health care disparities can be resolved.

1. Why is it important for health care workers and providers to be aware of their own biases when providing care to clients/patients?
2. Should higher education and schools offering diploma and certification training in health care fields of practice be held accountable for not educating their students about health disparities and discrimination in health care?

3. Why is it important to hold consumers in vulnerable populations accountable for their own health maintenance once documentation of risk factors and disease prevention has been completed by health care providers and a signed care plan is mutually developed?
4. Is it necessary for states and government programs to effectively use existing health disparity data to improve the quality of health care delivered in the US? If yes, explain why. If you disagree, explain why.
5. Is health care for diseases like Alzheimer's impacted by health disparities?

CASE STUDY: IS THERE A SOLUTION TO HEALTH DISPARITIES?

I get tired sometimes of going to health care professionals who do not even understand who I am or care to get to know me. I feel uncomfortable the moment I am not greeted by the receptionist at the desk. She makes brief eye contact and then hands me a clipboard, kindly stating, "Here you go. Update these." I get angry, but I feel more sad than angry, when I see the same receptionist have a full conversation and laugh with other patients who look like her. By the time I get to see the doctor, I await the poor eye contact and stereotypes that flood the conversation. They do, and I barely can remember why I even made the appointment in the first place.

Figure 1. Clear pathways take time

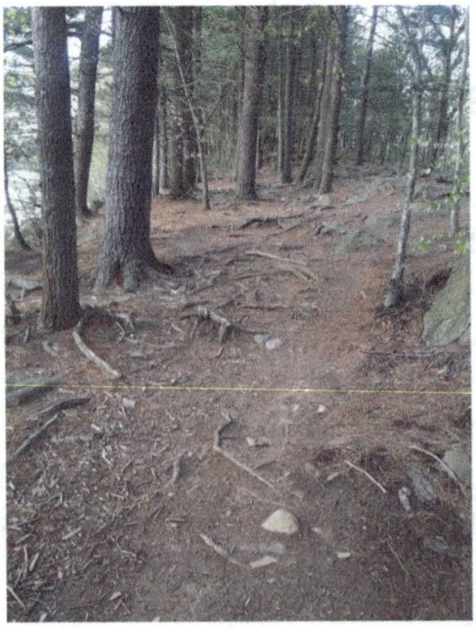

The doctor pauses, "Did you want more pain medication or something? Your blood pressure is good." I shake my head in silence and inform the doctor that I do not take any pain medications; I never have. He smiles and leaves the room. I sit quietly for a moment. Looks like it's time to find another new doctor.

Discussion: What made the client/patient feel uncomfortable and consider the need to secure a new health care provider?

REFERENCES

Alliance for Human Research and Protection. (2020). *1962: Dr. Chester Southam injected live cancer cells into 22 elderly patients.* https://ahrp.org/1962-dr-chester-southam-injected-live-cancer-cells-into-22-elderly-patients-at-jewish-chronic-disease-hospital-in-brooklyn/

Beecher, H. K. (1966). Ethics and clinical research. *The New England Journal of Medicine*, *274*(24), 1354–1360. doi:10.1056/NEJM196606162742405 PMID:5327352

Berger, R. L. (1990). Nazi science: The Dachau hypothermia experiments. *The New England Journal of Medicine*, *322*(20), 1435–1440. doi:10.1056/NEJM199005173222006 PMID:2184357

Brandt, A. M. (1978). Racism and research: The case of the Tuskegee syphilis study. *The Hastings Center Report*, *8*(6), 21–29. doi:10.2307/3561468 PMID:721302

Centers for Disease Control and Prevention. (2008). *Community Health and Program Services (CHAPS): Health disparities among racial/ethnic populations.* United States Department of Health and Human Services.

Centers for Disease Control and Prevention. (2019). *About chronic diseases.* https://www.cdc.gov/chronicdisease/about/index.htm

Centers for Disease Control and Prevention. (2020). *National Center for Chronic Disease Prevention and Health Promotion: Health and economic costs of chronic diseases.* https://www.cdc.gov/chronicdisease/about/costs/index.htm

Constantin, A. (2018). Human subject research: International and regional human rights standards. *Health and Human Rights Journal, 20*(2), 137–148. https://www.ncbi.nlm.nih.gov/pmc/articles/PMC6293356/

Grossman, S. C., & Porth, C. M. (2014). *Pathophysiology: Concepts of altered health states* (9th ed.). Lippincott Williams & Wilkins.

Harris, J. R. (2005). Social behavior and personality development: The role of experiences with siblings and with peers. In B. J. Ellis & D. F. Bjorklund (Eds.), *Origins of the social mind: Evolutionary psychology and child development* (pp. 245–270). Guilford Press.

Healthypeople.gov. (2020). *Secretary's Advisory Committee on National Health Promotion and Disease Prevention objectives for 2030.* https://www.healthypeople.gov/2020/About-Healthy-People/Development-Healthy-People-2030/Advisory-Committee

Hershey, G. A., & Miller, R. (1976). Human experimentation and the law. Academic Press.

Hinkle, J. L., & Cheever, K. H. (2018). *Brunner & Suddarth: Textbook of medical-surgical nursing* (14th ed.). Wolters Kluwer.

Justice, D. (2020). *The closing of Willowbrook: New York State Association for Retarded Children v. Carey.* https://disabilityjustice.org/the-closing-of-willowbrook/

Lattal, K. A., & Yoshioka, M. (2017). Improving the human instrument. *Revista Mexicana de Análisis de la Conducta, 43*(2), 177–191. doi:10.5514/rmac.v43.i2.62312

Levine, R. J. (1986). *Ethics and regulation of clinical research* (2nd ed.). Urban & Schwarzenberg.

Medicaid.gov. (2020a). *Financial management.* https://www.medicaid.gov/medicaid/financial-management/index.html

Medicaid.gov. (2020b). *March 2020 Medicaid & CHIP enrollment data highlights.* https://www.medicaid.gov/medicaid/program-information/medicaid-and-chip-enrollment-data/report-highlights/index.html

Medicare.gov. (2020). *How is Medicare funded?* https://www.medicare.gov/about-us/how-is-medicare-funded

Ross, W. D. (2002). *The right and the good.* Oxford University Press. (Original work published 1930) doi:10.1093/0199252653.001.0001

Rothman, D. J. (1982). Were Tuskegee and Willowbrook "studies in nature?". *The Hastings Center Report, 12*(2), 5–7. doi:10.2307/3561798 PMID:7096065

Steinfels, P., & Levine, C. (1976). Biomedical ethics and the shadow of Nazism. *The Hastings Center Report, 614*(4), 1–20. doi:10.2307/3560386 PMID:11678142

United States Department of Health and Human Services, Office of Human Research Protections. (2010). *Pre-2018 requirements.* https://www.hhs.gov/ohrp/regulations-and-policy/regulations/regulatory-text/index.html

United States Department of Health and Human Services, Office of Human Research Protections. (2019). *Revised common rule regulatory text.* https://www.hhs.gov/ohrp/regulations-and-policy/regulations/revised-common-rule-regulatory-text/index.html

Waisel, D. B. (2013). Vulnerable population in healthcare. *Current Opinion in Anaesthesiology, 26*(2), 186–192. doi:10.1097/ACO.0b013e32835e8c17 PMID:23385323

Weindling, P. (2005). Medicine and the Nuremberg Trials: From medical war crimes to informed consent. *British Medical Journal, 331*(7513), 408. doi:10.1136/bmj.331.7513.408

Chapter 7
Grassroots Community Collaboratives

ABSTRACT

Grassroots community initiatives can be vital to the education and stabilization of vulnerable populations experiencing problems, such as chronic disease and socioeconomic issues. A historical overview of the origins of some grassroots initiatives in the United States are explored. The potential effectiveness of grassroots initiatives used in the past and implemented in the current healthcare environment is examined for purposeful use in resolving health disparities. While, historically, there have been multiple interventions to resolve the problem of health disparities, the problem of socioeconomic and racial injustices still prevent change. Nonetheless, change is possible and can be accomplished.

LEARNING OBJECTIVES

1. Explain how grassroots movements have historically contributed to societal changes.
2. Explain how the New Deal did not alleviate the societal problem of health disparities.
3. Discuss how grassroots movements, like Cost-Offset Community Supported Agriculture (CO-CSA) programs, expanded to all Americans can improve health outcomes.

DOI: 10.4018/978-1-7998-3874-6.ch007

Reflection Quote: "I can confidently create change in my local community by starting a grassroots movement."

INTRODUCTION

A **grassroots movement** consists of the organization of people around a collective action whereby change is deemed necessary. Historically, there have been several grassroots movements within the US that have eventually led to the formulation of policies, regulations, and laws. Examples include the civil rights movement, women's suffrage movement, progressive movement (addressing labor protections, among other issues), and the formation of labor unions. Grassroots movements that emphasized health emerged in the early 20th century when ill Americans who were unable to work lost days from work, impacting the economy. Trattner (1989), in his discussion of the public health movement of the mid-19th century, described American cities as unsanitary, disease-ridden, and foul-smelling. Drainage systems were unable to accommodate garbage, and animal waste was strewn throughout cities. Diseases such as scarlet fever, cholera, typhus, diphtheria, tuberculosis, and smallpox threatened the lives of Americans living in crowded cities.

With the **Great Depression** (a worldwide economic recession that occurred during the 1930s), Hoffman (2003) noted that marches held by unemployed veterans, farmers, the elderly, and others led to the development of the New Deal. The **New Deal**, a set of policies passed by Congress and promoted by President Franklin D. Roosevelt between 1933 and 1939, was instrumental in helping the US emerge from the Great Depression. Other programs established by the US government include the Medicaid and Medicare programs, enacted in 1965.

Grassroots movements continue to evolve, with health care often taking center stage. With regard to health disparities, grassroots initiatives can be developed in affected communities through the empowerment of the community members themselves. Existing community-based clinics and healthcare systems can offer programs to affected communities in close proximity to them, with the focused goal of reducing risk factors associated with chronic disease development. The community-based clinics and healthcare systems would be required to document and show evidence of community members' sustained engagement to validate consumer accountability (see Chapter 6) of buy-in to improve their own health status.

Example of a Grassroots Initiative: Obesity

The World Health Organization (WHO) defines being obese and overweight as having an abnormal accumulation of fat that, in excess, poses a health risk. Persons with a body mass index (BMI) of more than 30 kg/m^2 are considered obese, and those with a BMI greater than 25 kg/m^2 are considered overweight. Chronic diseases, such as cancer, diabetes, and cardiovascular diseases, are more likely to occur in persons who are obese or overweight (WHO, 2020).

Obesity is a costly and serious disease that decreases the life span of affected adults, and its prevalence varies slightly. For adults 60 years and older, the prevalence is 42.8%; among middle-aged adults, 40–59 years, the prevalence is 44.8%; among young adults, 20–39 years, the prevalence is 40.0%. The prevalence of obesity in the US from 1999 to 2018 increased from 30.5% to 42.4%, and for severe obesity, it increased from 4.7% to 9.2%. In 2008, the annual medical cost associated with obesity was $147 billion. Obesity rates among different racial and ethnic groups include: non-Hispanic Asians (17.4%), non-Hispanic Whites (42.2%), Hispanics (44.8%), and non-Hispanic Blacks (49.6%). Variations in obesity rates have been associated with income, education, and race/ethnicity (CDC, 2020).

Zamora-Kapoor et al. (2019), in a systematic review of the literature addressing risk factors and the prevalence of obesity among American Indians and Alaska Natives, found that this population has the highest obesity prevalence in the US. The risk factors coincide with current identified risk factors, such as cardiovascular disease and diabetes (Boccuti, 2015; CDC, 2020), all of which increase with the presence of obesity. More research is needed to address obesity in the American Indian and Alaska Native populations. A grassroots initiative addressing obesity must include culturally informed education on nutrition, stress reduction, risk reduction for chronic disease, exercise, and education on socioeconomic implications for maintaining a healthy diet and making healthy food selections.

Example of a Grassroot Initiative: Nutrition

Nutrition is instrumental in disease prevention. Healthy lifestyles integrate nutrition in the maintenance of BMI, glycemic control, lowered cholesterol levels, and wound healing, among many other benefits. **Cost-Offset Community Supported Agriculture** (CO-CSA) programs are a means to introduce healthy foods from local farmers to low-income households. Participants in CO-CSA programs receive subsidized shares from the harvests of the farmers.

Garner et al. (2020) examined data from Washington, New York, Vermont, and North Carolina (n = 305) on CO-CSA programs presented in conjunction with a nutritional education component. Data were compared to the National Health and Nutrition Examination Survey conducted between 2007 and 2010. Participants were low-income adults with children within their households. Descriptive statistics were calculated for nutrition, demographics, and nutrition knowledge. The findings showed that the majority of participants in the CO-CSA programs were highly educated (49% versus 7% college graduates), White (76% versus 45%) females enrolled in the program (97% versus 57%) who experienced food insecurities (57% versus 49%). A small percentage of the females were Hispanic (6% versus 34%). CO-CSA participants were knowledgeable about the nutritional benefits of food, such as the recommendation of consuming 3–5 cups of vegetables and fruits per day (61% versus 16%), and reported having excellent or good health (34% versus 25%).

The CO-CSA program is an excellent example of how existing programs can be expanded to include low-income diverse populations throughout the US. Learning about healthy foods and the benefits of nutrition in disease prevention, can save lives. If each of the 50 states and the District of Columbia, as well as the US territories, were required to adopt and maintain the CO-CSA program for low-income Americans, this could be another means of decreasing health disparity.

SUMMARY

Grassroots initiatives can be implemented within communities through collaboration with community members and health care organizations, and state, local, and federal governments to improve health disparities. Successful programs should target risk factors associated with chronic disease prevention, such as smoking cessation, nutrition, access to healthy water, reduction of community-based sources of pollutants (i.e., dumps), or improvement of old, dilapidated school buildings. Change is not always equated with power, but its outcome should be empowerment.

GRASSROOTS CHANGE

Directions: Review each statement and question. Contemplate how grassroots movements can lead to changes in health care that could decrease or eliminate health inequities.

1. Identify at least four community-based grassroots initiatives that can be developed that impact health disparities in the US.
2. What grassroots initiative can a small community-based hospital implement to prevent high rates of food poisoning in local restaurants that have occurred over the course of one month?
3. Why is it important for community members to participate in grassroots initiatives in their own neighborhoods?
4. Do all grassroots initiatives require finances to be successful? Provide an example.
5. Why are community gardens a good grassroots initiative to start in urban and rural communities?
6. What could be the benefit of a grassroots initiative to promote a walking group for retired seniors over the age of 65 years?
7. Consider a grassroots initiative that can be started to reduce the number of maternal deaths of African American women in the US. Whom should the initiative involve?
8. Should community-based churches or schools be involved in grassroots initiatives impacting families within their communities? If yes, what kind of initiatives?

CASE STUDY: "I CAN MAKE A CHANGE."

I live in a **food desert**. There are more liquor stores and fast-food restaurants in my neighborhood than there are grocery stores. And the grocery stores sell sodas and juices that have 10% juice and 90% high fructose corn syrup. I can easily buy low-cost frozen and canned foods loaded with salt, but there are limited amounts of fresh fruits and vegetables.

My diabetes was out of control, and my blood pressure was too. I was excited to read about how some communities, with the permission of their city or town, had developed gardens that fed entire communities. I went from house to house asking for volunteers in my neighborhood to work with me on the garden and before I knew it, I had 25 people.

The community garden has been in existence now for two years. My diabetes is under control and I no longer have high blood pressure. I am also very close to my neighbors, and we have successfully advocated for a healthy grocery store to be built in our neighborhood. Sometimes it just takes one person to make positive change and end health disparities.

Discussion: Can programs developed in local communities to address health disparities be successfully expanded to counties?

Figure 1. Pathways

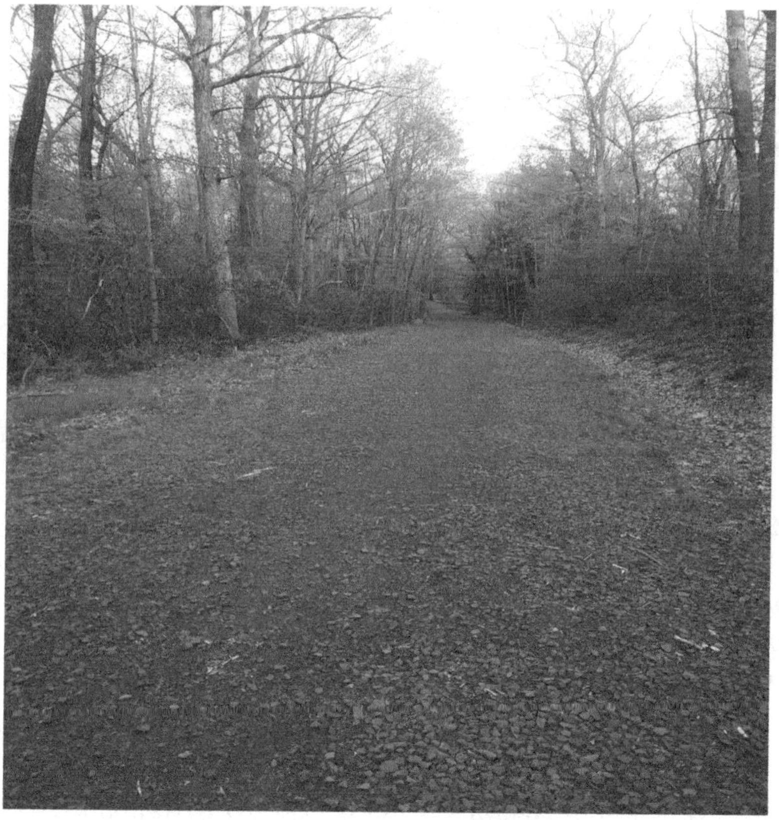

REFERENCES

Boccuti, C. L. (2015). Chronic disease and limited access to healthcare still beset American Indians and Alaska Natives. *Aging Today*, *32*(2), 5–13. https://www.asaging.org/blog/chronic-disease-and-limited-access-healthcare-still-beset-american-indians-and-alaska-natives

Centers for Disease Control and Prevention. (2020). *Overweight and obesity: Adult obesity facts*. https://www.cdc.gov/obesity/data/adult.html

Centers for Medicare and Medicaid Services. (2020). *History: CMS program history*. https://www.cms.gov/About-CMS/Agency-Information/History

Garner, J., Lepior, H., Taylor, C., Hanson, K., Ammerman, A., Pitts, S. J., Kolondinsky, J., Sitaker, M., & Seguin-Fowler, R. (2020). P78 low-income adults enrolled in a cost-offset, community supported agriculture intervention are not nationally representative. *Journal of Nutrition Education and Behavior*, *52*(7), S53. doi:10.1016/j.jneb.2020.04.124 PMID:31924558

Hoffman, B. (2003). Health care reform and social movements in the United States. *American Journal of Public Health*, *93*(1), 75–85. doi:10.2105/AJPH.93.1.75 PMID:12511390

Medicaid.gov. (2020). *Program history*. https://www.medicaid.gov/about-us/program-history/index.html

Trattner, W. I. (1989). *From poor law to welfare state: A history of social welfare in America* (4th ed.). The Free Press.

World Health Organization. (2020). *Health topics: Obesity. Garner et al. (2020) examined data from Washington, New York, Vermont, and North Carolina (n = 305) on CO-CSA programs Garner et al. (2020) examined data from Washington, New York, Vermont, and North Carolina (n = 305) on CO-CSA programs*. https://www.who.int/topics/obesity/en/

Zamora-Kapoor, A., Sinclair, K., Nelson, L., Lee, H., & Buchwald, D. (2019). Obesity risk factors in American Indians and Alaskan Natives: A systematic review. *Public Health*, *174*, 85–96. doi:10.1016/j.puhe.2019.05.021 PMID:31326761

Chapter 8
Holding Healthcare Systems Accountable

ABSTRACT

Statistically, there are data that support the persistent existence of health disparities in the United States. Should healthcare systems and facilities be held accountable by their state and the federal government to show evidence of improvements in recognizing and resolving disparities experienced by vulnerable populations receiving care within their organizations? The answer to this question is yes. If healthcare systems consistently produce data indicative of poor health outcomes for vulnerable populations, interventions should be identified to improve healthcare delivery and quality. Improvements in the health status of all Americans is contingent upon a united front by all Americans in ending health disparities.

LEARNING OBJECTIVES

1. Explain why it is important to hold healthcare systems accountable for health disparities and inequities that occur within their facilities?
2. Compare and contrast situations that can impact patients' engagement in health care when healthcare providers and workers lack insight into patients' cultural expectations.
3. Explain why it is important for patients to understand their diagnoses and how to manage acute and chronic diseases.

DOI: 10.4018/978-1-7998-3874-6.ch008

4. Discuss the necessity of empowering patients with questions and statements to ask healthcare providers so that they can become proactive in their treatment regimen.

Reflection Quote: "I feel like I can take better care of myself whenever I learn something new about my condition. It makes me feel empowered."

INTRODUCTION

The engagement of vulnerable populations in community-based initiatives is imperative to the reduction of health disparities. Community-based initiatives can involve ethical research collaborations with vulnerable populations and the health systems that serve them. By engaging and establishing trust with vulnerable populations that have high rates of health disparities in the US, genomic studies (Hull, 2019) can be implemented and identification of lifestyle and treatment modifications investigated, for the reduction and elimination of health disparities. The World Health Organization (WHO) defines **genomics** as "the study of genes and their functions, and related techniques" (WHO, 2002, 2004, 2021). Meanwhile, **genetics** examines the composition and function of a single gene. Comparatively, genomics examines the relationships of genes to identify the genes' combined effects on the development and growth of an organism (WHO, 2021).

INJECTION DRUG USE AMONG ALASKA NATIVES AND AMERICAN INDIANS

Leston et al. (2018) conducted a community-based study to identify steps that could be taken to reduce health disparities for American Indians and Alaska Natives who inject drugs. The goal was to increase knowledge on the importance of preventing the hepatitis C virus and human immunodeficiency virus (HIV), and build sustainable health programs in tribal communities. Collaboration in the research process between tribal members and researchers assisting in the community-based initiative was instrumental to the planning and implementation processes.

Therapeutically, opioids are prescribed to reduce pain. Nationally, opioid use disorders have increased throughout the US (AMA, 2013). Since 1999, more than 750,000 people have died from drug overdoses. In 2018, two out of three drug overdoses involving opioids included drugs such as fentanyl (a synthetic opioid), heroin, or prescription opioids (CDC, 2020). However, data specific to American Indian and Alaska Natives regarding opioid use disorders is limited (Leston et al., 2018).

Research participants were recruited from four tribal communities that were culturally and geographically diverse. Thirty-two interviews were completed with persons who either had a history of injecting drugs or who were actively injecting drugs. From the interviews, five themes were identified that could impact the implementation of the community-based program, including: structure, innovation, patient, organizational, and provider. Factors impacting the five themes were explored in terms of how they could affect policy-making (Leston et al., 2018).

In reviewing the five interview themes, *innovation* examined overdosing being witnessed or having been experienced by the tribal member(s). Tribal members were unaware of existing partnerships with law enforcement, schools, tribal governments, and non-profit organizations to provide resources to address injection drug use in the community. Ideas for implementing the theme of *innovation* were to ensure the enactment of **Good Samaritan laws**—under which a person is protected from legal claims of negligence if they provide care to someone in an emergency situation in absence of the expectation of being paid—at the tribal level and community-wide education (Leston et al., 2018; West & Varacallo, 2020).

The *patient* theme explored risk-taking behaviors versus protective behaviors by persons who injected drugs, such as needle sharing and unhygienic injecting. The impact of addiction was an area identified as needing more awareness by the tribal communities. Withdrawing from others, social isolation, the contraction of disease, drug withdrawal, and physical responses to addiction were identified as reasons why affected tribal members did not seek addiction treatment. An implication for implementing the theme of *patient* was recognition of the need for the tribes to ensure that they engaged with behavioral health services for addiction treatment (Leston et al., 2018).

Healthcare *provider* interactions were reported by participants as being both negative—whereby they felt judged and stigmatized—and positive—when healthcare providers were non-judgmental and demonstrated compassion. Overall, providers were viewed as needing more training to understand how to support persons who injected drugs and addiction. Cultural competency by healthcare providers working with tribal members was also an area identified as needing improvement. Implications for implementing the healthcare provider theme focused on provider education and on tribal members and healthcare providers being open to new attitudes, practice approaches, and evidenced-based practices associated with working with persons who inject drugs (Leston et al., 2018).

The *organizational* theme explored perceptions of services versus available resources. Each of the four tribes geographically varied in terms of the services available to treat persons with addictions involving the injection of drugs. An implication for the *organizational* theme for tribal members was that there needed to be more programs to address addiction that were culturally competent (Leston et al., 2018).

Lastly, the *structural* theme examined barriers encountered by persons in obtaining clean needles. Pharmacy store hours, prescription requirements, scarcity of funds for needle programs, and societal labels used by healthcare providers and tribal community members were identified as barriers. Policies for harm reduction, treatment services, and fear of being reported to law enforcement all resulted in persons who injected drugs having difficulty seeking sobriety. Implications for the implementation of the *structural* theme were that tribal members and the state in which the tribe(s) reside must increase awareness of available resources, avoid the criminalization of paraphernalia (needles), and promote help-seeking behaviors for persons who inject drugs (Leston et al., 2018).

When people have historically been marginalized in society, trust is lost and replaced with suspicion. It is imperative that researchers collaborate with tribal communities to discuss their health disparities and use genomic research to examine health disparities (Hull, 2019). Ultimately, the goal is to decrease and eliminate one health disparity at a time.

LOW-INCOME POPULATIONS AND CANCER HEALTH DISPARITIES

In 2014, cancer mortality rates among low-income populations were higher than those of heart disease (Heron & Anderson, 2016). The latter was noted in 22 of the 50 states (Heron & Anderson, 2016). National hearings addressing how cancer negatively impacts low-income populations were hosted by the American Cancer Society in seven cities in 1989 (American Cancer Society, 1989). Access to preventive health care, such as annual physicals with healthcare providers, requires the poor to have adequate insurance coverage.

The poor also benefit from programs that teach the benefits of eating healthy foods and maintaining a BMI that is not equated with being overweight or obese; all factors contributed to cancer diagnoses.

A criticism of cancer education programs is that they tend to not be culturally sensitive (Calhoun, 2017). These programs are also not often made available in areas where vulnerable populations reside. Other factors are occupational hazards (i.e., exposures to chemicals, dust, etc.), tobacco use, food insecurity, alcohol intake, and inadequate housing and chronic diseases (i.e., diabetes) that are poorly managed, further compromising general health status prior to a cancer diagnosis.

TEACHING VULNERABLE POPULATIONS TO ADVOCATE FOR THEMSELVES IN HEALTHCARE ENVIRONMENTS

All People Deserve Quality Care

When discussing health care in the US, the conversation must include that all people have the right to receive quality health care that is evidence based. The delivery of this care should be from competent providers who have been taught that implicit biases exist. However, once unconscious biases, including stereotypes of other groups, are brought to consciousness, the professional expectation is that health care is to be delivered with the realization that *all people deserve quality care*. Quality health care delivered to all people despite their sex, age, religion, race, ethnicity, or culture, is non-negotiable.

Understanding the Basics of Healthcare Systems

Healthcare systems are comprised of different people in positions (e.g. respiratory therapists, social workers, chaplains, psychologists, physicians, nurses, physical therapists, dieticians, occupational therapists, and speech pathologist, etc.) that provide the service of healing to persons whose health has become physiologically and psychologically compromised. Illness, injury, pathological and physiological diseases, and stress can contribute to the decline in the health of all humans. Hence, understanding how to navigate healthcare systems is imperative in protecting one's health.

Healthcare systems can include hospitals, emergency departments, chaplaincy departments, clinics (e.g., optometry, orthotics, medical, cardiac, and surgical, etc.), and outpatient services that are specialized, such as mental health, diabetes management, chemotherapy infusion centers (for patients being treated for cancer), podiatry (foot care/lower extremities), palliative care, and offices for several healthcare providers (e.g., physicians, nurse practitioners, and PAs) that provide care to people entering the healthcare system for services.

Why Are Healthcare Systems Necessary?

Healthcare systems are necessary because they can effectively serve densely populated areas requiring access to multiple services (i.e., specialty clinics, rehabilitation services, comprehensive laboratory and diagnostic services, and academic healthcare providers who are experts in their fields of practice and study) for varied health care problems. Additionally, healthcare systems that have purchased smaller community hospitals and facilities (i.e., long-term care or rehabilitation facilities) can immediately extend these services to towns and rural areas that would otherwise be unable to meet the complex needs of the populations they serve. Healthcare systems, because of their large size and multiple sources of income, are more likely to have innovative technologies and evidence-based treatment modalities available.

Routine Annual Exams and As-Needed Healthcare providers

In healthcare providers' offices there are different providers who can examine patients to determine a diagnosis of illness or disease. Healthcare providers include **advanced practice registered nurses (APRNs)**, physicians, and **physician assistants (PAs).** PAs are trained in graduate programs to differentiate disease processes, physiological problems, and emotional or mental health problems. Practice areas for PAs vary based on the specializations selected (i.e., medicine, surgery, rehabilitation, psychiatry, substance abuse, orthopedics, etc.). PAs collaborate with other health care team members in the management and determination of diagnoses of patients. Additionally, PAs offer physical examinations that include patients' health histories, and they can order laboratory and diagnostic tests. PAs also prescribe medications and provide preventive health care. However, PAs must practice under the supervision of licensed physicians in all aspects of their clinical practice.

APRNs are registered nurses who attend graduate programs that reiterate at a higher level the diagnostic understanding of disease pathologies. Nurses advance from the assessment of patients to providing physical examinations. APRNs can order diagnostic and laboratory tests, prescribe medications, provide preventive health care, and work in specializations like PAs. However, APRNs can independently practice clinically in office settings in absence of a physician.

Physicians attend medical school and must complete extensive residency programs based on their specializations. While PAs and APRNs also have residency programs, requirements may vary by state in terms of what clinical practices are allowed, such as prescribing certain medications (i.e., narcotics). Physicians can treat injuries and illnesses, and diagnose disease processes. Physicians can also offer consultation on preventive health care, dietary modifications, and hygiene care to prevent infection. Additionally, physicians complete physical examinations and medical histories, interpret laboratory and diagnostic tests, and prescribe medications.

How Should I Prepare for My Visit With a Healthcare provider?

In preparation for a visit to see a healthcare provider, it is important for persons to organize their information that is to be shared during the visit. In doing so, no information is forgotten and healthcare providers can develop a potential diagnosis or treat an illness or injury effectively. Examples of information that can be given to healthcare providers include:

1. A list of all current medications;
2. A list of past medications prescribed within the period of one to two years;
3. Current symptoms that led to the visit;
4. Allergies to drugs, foods, or the environment;
5. Seasonal allergies;
6. Use of oxygen therapy, particularly if intermittent;
7. Frequency and type of physical exercise engaged in weekly;
8. Example of dietary intake of foods and beverages in the course of 48 to 72 hours;
9. Blood glucose levels over a period of at least one week if a diabetic;
10. Presence of pain or discomfort, location, triggers, longevity, degree of discomfort and pain;

11. Gastrointestinal problems (e.g., nausea, vomiting, gastroesophageal reflux disease, bloating, changes in bowel patterns, including diarrhea or constipation and blood in the stool), and abdominal pain;
12. Reproductive history;
13. Number of sexual partners;
14. Contraceptive use;
15. Gender;
16. Sexual identity and sexual practices with intimate partners;
17. Domestic violence or history of domestic violence;
18. Safety in the home;
19. Number of children within the home, if relevant;
20. Number of supportive adults in the home (i.e., potential caregivers);
21. Presence of refrigeration;
22. Presence of pets within the home;
23. Presence of air conditioners or heating units;
24. Any skin issues, such as reddened areas, rashes, pimples, moles, or wounds that are healing slowly (or draining pus);
25. Easily bruising skin;
26. Joint, muscle, or bone pain;
27. Headaches;
28. Blurry vision, double vision, pain in the eyes, narrowed vision, or bloodshot eyes;
29. Elevated blood pressure;
30. Low blood pressure;
31. Dizziness;
32. Blood in the stool or urine;
33. Painful urination or narrowed stream;
34. Difficulty having a bowel movement;
35. Difficulty emptying the bladder or feeling full after urinating;
36. Loss of teeth, cavities, abscesses, or sores in the mouth;
37. Nose bleeds;
38. Heavy menstrual cycles or irregular menstrual cycles;
39. Decreased libidos;
40. Ear pain or drainage;
41. Nasal discomfort or frequent or new presentation of nasal drainage;
42. A recent fall or injury to any part of the body;
43. A recent injury to the head sustained by a blow to the head or a fall;
44. Histories of cardiac or respiratory problems;
45. Compromised mobility requiring the use of an assistive device;

46. Hair loss or brittle hair;
47. Nail fungus, change in nail thickness, nail clubbing, nail coloration changes, or presence of striae;
48. Cold hands;
49. Variations in body warmth or coolness;
50. Dry skin or skin that is cool and clammy;
51. Skin that flakes or tears easily;
52. Jaw pain;
53. Recent laboratory tests;
54. Recent diagnostic tests;
55. Preventive care, laboratory and diagnostics (for prostate cancer, prostatitis, or benign prostatic hyperplasia—males—and breast cancer, mammography, or ultrasound for dense breast tissue—females);
56. Hormone levels for testosterone, progesterone, and estrogen;
57. Back pain;
58. Knee pain;
59. Arm pain;
60. Neck pain;
61. Chest pain;
62. Changes in speech, including slurring and hoarseness;
63. Difficulty in remembering recent or remote life events;
64. Alcohol intake;
65. Smoking history;
66. Illegal and legal drug use or abuse;
67. Use of psychiatric medications;
68. Recent visit to see a therapist or counselor;
69. Foul-smelling or fruity-smelling breath;
70. Tender sinuses around the face;
71. Swollen glands (e.g., around the neck, axillary areas, etc.);
72. Fevers;
73. Frequent cough;
74. Productive cough;
75. Shoulder pain;
76. Projectile vomiting;
77. Inflammation around joints and redness;
78. Colonoscopy to rule out colon cancer;
79. Inquire about laboratory tests to ensure that there are no issues with electrolytes, kidney, or liver functioning;
80. Irregular heartbeats or palpitations;

81. Anxiety, depression, or auditory or visual hallucinations;
82. Drainage from the nipples, dimpling, or presence of open sores;
83. Unexplained fatigue;
84. Pale palms or oral cavity indicative of anemia;
85. History of abortion(s);
86. Religion and faith; and
87. Cultural and ethnic background.

In the management of acute and chronic conditions, it is important for patients to use available resources to gain knowledge about their diseases. By gaining knowledge about diagnosed diseases and other health issues, patients are empowered and can better provide self-care. Disease management is imperative to maintaining health and longevity of life. Below are some examples of websites that patients can access to learn how to care for themselves and successfully manage their health:

- American Diabetes Association- https://www.diabetes.org/
- American Cancer Society- https://www.cancer.org/
- American Society for Metabolic and Bariatric Surgery- https://asmbs.org/
- National Cancer Institute- https://www.cancer.gov/
- Cancer Information (Medline Plus)- https://www.nlm.nih.gov/medlineplus/cancer.html
- Organ Transplantation (Medline Plus)- https://www.nlm.nih.gov/medlineplus/organtransplantation.html
- National Stroke Association- https://www.stroke.org/American Spinal Injury Association- https://asia-spinalinjury.org/
- Epilepsy Foundation- https://www.epilepsy.com/
- Epilepsy Foundation of Connecticut- https://www.epilepsyct.com/
- American Heart Association- https://www.heart.org/HEARTORG/
- American Burn Association- https://ameriburn.org/

SUMMARY

Solutions to health care disparities must involve healthcare systems and other facilities and providers who work with vulnerable populations. Communities that have vulnerable populations that have documented health disparities should require health care organizations that provide services in the community to record data on identified health disparities. Additionally, clinical measurement instruments can be secured to gather data focused on health promotion and the alleviation of health disparities while also using data to decipher if equitable resolution of disparities is occurring.

It is imperative that patients be regularly provided evidence-based resources in their native language on their diagnosed disease processes. This information should be provided both verbally and in writing to ensure thoroughness and accuracy of content delivery. Additionally, the Internet can be used to provide patients with information on support groups, dietary interventions, current research, exercise, physiological and psychological changes, and medications and treatment interventions. A thorough educational session can also bring to healthcare providers' and workers' awareness patients' financial constraints in complying with their treatment regimens (e.g., medication and medical equipment purchases). Empowering patients with information regarding the management of their diseases can help decrease health disparities.

Figure 1. Patient Empowerment

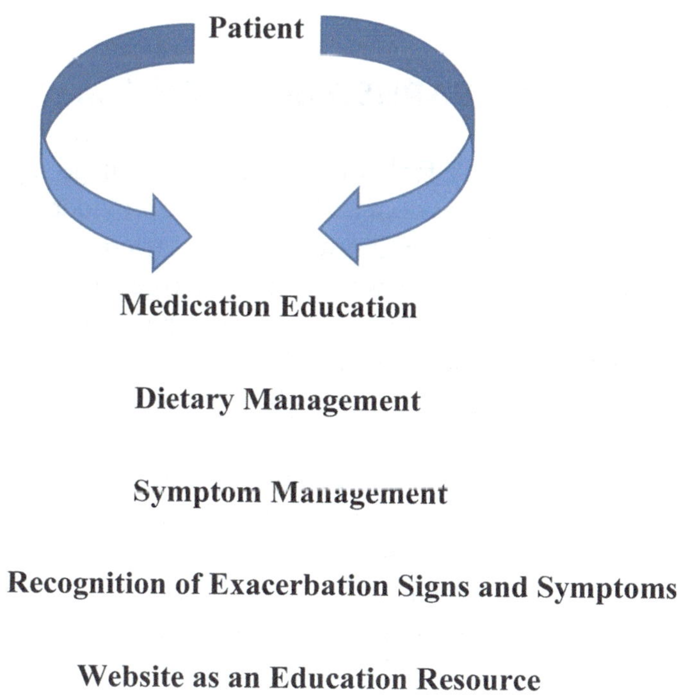

HEALTHCARE SYSTEM ACCOUNTABILITY

Directions: Read each question about healthcare system accountability and consider whether organizations and facilities should be held accountable for health disparities. Should there be more research monies dedicated to health disparities and inequities faced by Americans in our current healthcare systems?

1. Why should healthcare systems demonstrate accountability in their community-based care of vulnerable populations residing near their facilities?
2. Why is it important for healthcare systems to record health disparity data within their zone of operation?
3. Should health care organizations be fined by their state for not addressing health disparities in the populations they regularly serve?
4. Should health care organizations be seen as a profit-making industry only? In other words, should they be understood as having no moral obligation to the people to whom they provide health care other than to ensure that the care delivered is evidence based, of quality, and safe?

CASE STUDY: "I'VE LEARNED SO MUCH."

After all these years, I finally feel smart enough to manage my diabetes. I honestly did not know what I was doing. My healthcare provider just prescribed the tablets and assumed all was going well. When I tried to ask questions, I felt rushed and that the expectation was low for me to get better or understand how to improve my health care. I was discouraged and depressed.

I could not believe it when my healthcare provider came in one day and explained to me that he had taken a class on implicit bias and cultural sensitivity. He looked at me and said, "Do you understand how to keep your blood glucose levels lowered?" I was so relieved and shook my head, "No." He then took out a piece of paper and started to explain to me how insulin worked in my body, along with the importance of diet and exercise. It was the best time I ever had in a healthcare provider's office!

I felt heard and understood. In just two months, I lost weight, my diabetes numbers were within normal limits, and I felt like a younger person. My healthcare provider and I have a great relationship now, and I am healthier.

Discussion: What helped this patient be able to better manage their diabetes?

Figure 2. Pathways continue

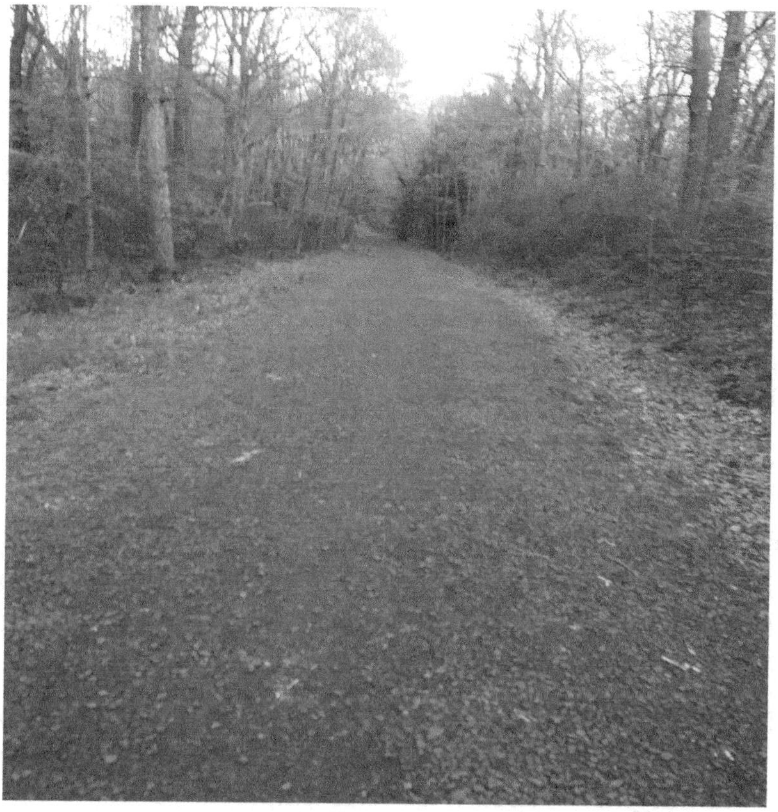

REFERENCES

American Cancer Society. (1989). *A summary of the American Cancer Society report to the nation: Cancer in the poor*. https://acsjournals.onlinelibrary.wiley.com/doi/pdf/10.3322/canjclin.39.5.263

American Psychiatric Association. (2013). *Desk reference to the diagnostic criteria from DSM-5*. American Psychiatric Publishing.

Calhoun, D. (2017). Cancer health disparities among low-income populations. *Journal of Oncology Navigation & Survivorship*, *8*(1), 38–39.

Centers for Disease Control and Prevention. (2020). *Data overview. The drug overdose epidemic: Behind the numbers*. https://www.cdc.gov/drugoverdose/data/index.html

Heron, M., & Anderson, R. N. (2016). *Changes in the leading cause of death: Recent patterns in heart disease and cancer mortality*. https://www.cdc.gov/nchs/data/databriefs/db254.pdf

Hull, S. C. (2019). Changing the conversation about the ethics of genomics and health disparities research with American Indian and Alaska Native communities: A report from the field. *Journal of Health Care for the Poor and Underserved, 30*(4S), 21–26. doi:10.1353/hpu.2019.0111 PMID:31735714

Leston, J., Crisp, C., Lee, C., & Rink, E. (2018). An interview project with native American people: A community-based study to identify actionable steps to reduce health disparities. *Public Health, 176*, 82–91. doi:10.1016/j.puhe.2018.12.002 PMID:30765139

West, B., & Varacallo, M. (2020). *Good Samaritan laws*. Stat Pearls Publishing. https://www.ncbi.nlm.nih.gov/books/NBK542176/

World Health Organization. (2002). *Genomics and world health: Report of the Advisory Committee on Health Research, Geneva.* https://apps.who.int/iris/bitstream/handle/10665/42453/a74580.pdf;jsessionid=8688CBD365624947C31728322C08BE46?sequence=1

World Health Organization. (2004). *WHA 57. 13: Genomics and World Health, Fifty Seventh World Health Assembly Resolution*. https://apps.who.int/gb/ebwha/pdf_files/WHA57/A57_R13-en.pdf?ua=1

World Health Organization. (2021). *Human genomics in global health*. https://www.who.int/genomics/geneticsVSgenomics/en/#:~:text=Genomics%20is%20defined%20as%20the,their%20functions%2C%20and%20related%20techniques

APPENDIX

Exercises to Promote the Resolution of Health Disparities

Exercise 1. Introspection

A. Patients

If you feel uncomfortable sharing with your healthcare provider questions about your health, you may need to change providers or write a short list of prioritized concerns you have about your health and the indecisiveness you have regarding the continuation of the patient–provider relationship. Discuss your concerns with your provider. If there is no resolution, consider ending the patient–provider relationship. Never settle for less-than-optimal health care. By settling, you may shorten your life span. Health care loyalty is not one-sided when it comes to the patient–provider relationship.

It does not matter how long you have been a patient of your provider. Contact your insurance company and request a referral to a new provider. Call several providers and request to visit the healthcare provider's office and briefly meet the provider to ensure that the relationship is a good fit for your health care needs.

Exercises to Promote the Resolution of Health Disparities

Exercise 1. Introspection

B. Health Care Workers and Healthcare providers

Sometimes it can be difficult to take the time in a busy practice to talk with a patient. However, when that patient is of a different race and culture from your own, it is imperative that you learn how they understand your instructions in the management of their acute or chronic disease. Language barriers can further complicate patient instruction and understanding of how to follow medication and treatment regimens, and recognize the signs and symptoms of a worsening condition.

Teach patients by referencing learning methodologies. Inquire if your patients are visual, kinesthetic, or auditory learners. Provide materials that can meet patients' learning needs and use them to help patients understand their diagnoses. When patients feel that they can manage their own health care, they may be more likely to comply with your prescribed treatment regimens.

Exercises to Promote the Resolution of Health Disparities

Exercise 2: Humanness

A. Patients

It is important that patients understand that patient–provider and patient–health care worker relationships are not those of subordinate and authoritarian. Patients, when it comes to getting their health needs met in health care environments, must be equal participants in their health care plan. For example, that means that patients must remove all distractors, such as cutting off a television or radio, when health care team members enter their hospital room, and focus on what is being discussed about their own health care progression.

Bring a notebook to the office or hospital setting with a writing utensil and take notes. Ask about medication dosages prescribed, medication interactions, side effects, and the length of time you will have to be prescribed the medication to treat your condition. Inquire about the availability of alternative treatments and dietary and exercise regimens. Also ask about community-based support groups to learn more about your condition, and resources (i.e., financial or via a drug company or insurance) that can be accessed if needed to maintain disease management.

Exercises to Promote the Resolution of Health Disparities

Exercise 2: Humanness

B. Health Care Workers and Healthcare providers

Respect is a universal language that all humans speak. It is imperative that health care workers and providers be cognizant of the importance of being respectful in their interactions with all patients and one another. If there is awareness of the tendency to treat others without respect because of their sex, race, language, age, religion, or culture, this can be corrected with education on the part of the health care team to better serve affected populations with educational trainings on the prevention of health disparities and inequities.

Reflection Quote: "To bring unity and end hatred, we must reach to healing and forgiveness. Perhaps this is the only way that we, as a nation, can end health disparities and inequities."

Conclusion

Healthcare disparities among vulnerable populations can be resolved. The United States is a country rich with history embodied by diversity. Diversity and imperfections within humanity are normal. Physiologically and psychologically, variations in genetics and genomics is what causes *Homo sapiens*, as a species, to both thrive and survive. Racism and discrimination lead to our self-defeat and deteriorate our humanity, as they unnecessarily and illogically impact the health care of our fellow human beings.

Related Readings

To continue IGI Global's long-standing tradition of advancing innovation through emerging research, please find below a compiled list of recommended IGI Global book chapters and journal articles in the areas of healthcare disparities and solutions. These related readings will provide additional information and guidance to further enrich your knowledge and assist you with your own research.

A., D. R., Sharma, A. K., & Manikandan, A. (2020). Intra-Personal Emotional Intelligence Among College Students in Vellore District of Tamil Nadu. In *Innovations and Technologies for Soft Skill Development and Learning* (pp. 81-90). IGI Global. http://doi:10.4018/978-1-7998-3464-9.ch010

Abraham, J., Septian, D. L., Prayoga, T., & Ruman, Y. S. (2020). Predictive Factors of Attitude Towards Online Disruptive Advertising. In R. Leon (Ed.), *Strategies for Business Sustainability in a Collaborative Economy* (pp. 102–121). IGI Global. doi:10.4018/978-1-7998-4543-0.ch006

Adcock, A., Cram, F., & Lawton, B. (2019). E Hine. In D. Akella (Ed.), *Socio-Cultural Influences on Teenage Pregnancy and Contemporary Prevention Measures* (pp. 250–272). IGI Global. doi:10.4018/978-1-5225-6108-8.ch014

Ahmad, F., Wang, J. J., & El Morr, C. (2018). Online Mindfulness Interventions. In C. El Morr (Ed.), *Novel Applications of Virtual Communities in Healthcare Settings* (pp. 1–27). IGI Global. doi:10.4018/978-1-5225-2958-3.ch001

Ahuja, N. N. (2021). Yoga as a Complementary Therapy for ADHD. In R. T. Gopalan (Ed.), *New Developments in Diagnosing, Assessing, and Treating ADHD* (pp. 305–317). IGI Global. doi:10.4018/978-1-7998-5495-1.ch019

Akella, N. R. (2019). At the Mercy of Facebook. In D. Akella (Ed.), *Socio-Cultural Influences on Teenage Pregnancy and Contemporary Prevention Measures* (pp. 129–149). IGI Global. doi:10.4018/978-1-5225-6108-8.ch008

AlBarashdi, H. S., & Bouazza, A. (2019). Smartphone Usage, Gratifications, and Addiction. In X. Xu (Ed.), *Impacts of Mobile Use and Experience on Contemporary Society* (pp. 86–111). IGI Global. doi:10.4018/978-1-5225-7885-7.ch006

Aleksandrs, G. (2019). Working With Lesbian, Gay, Bisexual, and Transgender People in Care Relationships. In J. M. Martin (Ed.), *Mental Health Policy, Practice, and Service Accessibility in Contemporary Society* (pp. 177–204). IGI Global. doi:10.4018/978-1-5225-7402-6.ch010

Aleksić, V. (2020). Interactive TV. In D. Politis, P. Stagiopoulos, & V. Aleksić (Eds.), *Advanced Technologies and Standards for Interactive Educational Television* (pp. 206–212). IGI Global. doi:10.4018/978-1-7998-0253-2.ch010

Alkan, Ö., & Yarbaşı, İ. Y. (2020). Investigation of Alcohol Consumption Determinants in Turkey With Multinomial Probit Model. In S. Paul & S. Kulshreshtha (Eds.), *Global Developments in Healthcare and Medical Tourism* (pp. 134–161). IGI Global. doi:10.4018/978-1-5225-9787-2.ch008

Alvarez, L. (2018). Uberization of Healthcare. In V. E. Papalois & M. Theodosopoulou (Eds.), *Optimizing Health Literacy for Improved Clinical Practices* (pp. 87–93). IGI Global. doi:10.4018/978-1-5225-4074-8.ch005

Anderson, B. (2019). Revisiting MMORPGs in Support of Learning. In K. Becnel (Ed.), *Emerging Technologies in Virtual Learning Environments* (pp. 187–214). IGI Global. doi:10.4018/978-1-5225-7987-8.ch010

Andoh-Quainoo, L. (2020). Examining the Psychosocial Dimensions of Young People's Emergent Social Media Behavior. In M. Desjarlais (Ed.), *The Psychology and Dynamics Behind Social Media Interactions* (pp. 368–389). IGI Global. doi:10.4018/978-1-5225-9412-3.ch015

Andrews, U., Tarasenko, Y., & Holland, K. (2020). Complexities of Coordinating Service-Learning Experiences in Rural Communities. In U. Thomas (Ed.), *Cases on Strategic Partnerships for Resilient Communities and Schools* (pp. 192–210). IGI Global. doi:10.4018/978-1-7998-3285-0.ch012

Ansell, R. E., Morales, W. G., Kuras, A., Requa, C. M., & Mulvaney, T. (2021). Leading Transformational Experiences for K-8 Teachers. In L. N. Roberts (Ed.), *Redesigning Teaching, Leadership, and Indigenous Education in the 21st Century* (pp. 196–218). IGI Global. doi:10.4018/978-1-7998-5557-6.ch010

Aral, N., & Kadan, G. (2020). Technology and Teachers in the Preschool Period. In M. Durnali & İ. Limon (Eds.), *Enriching Teaching and Learning Environments With Contemporary Technologies* (pp. 221–240). IGI Global. doi:10.4018/978-1-7998-3383-3.ch013

Arble, E. P., & Arnetz, B. B. (2020). Evidence-Based Practices to Enhance First Responder Well-Being and Performance. In Mental Health Intervention and Treatment of First Responders and Emergency Workers (pp. 205-229). IGI Global. http://doi:10.4018/978-1-5225-9803-9.ch012

Arslan, G. (2019). Psychological Maltreatment and Digital Addiction. In B. Bozoglan (Ed.), *Multifaceted Approach to Digital Addiction and Its Treatment* (pp. 138–155). IGI Global. doi:10.4018/978-1-5225-8449-0.ch007

Arslan, Ü., & Kılınç, M. (2019). Important Factors in Vocational Decision-Making Process. In T. Fidan (Ed.), *Vocational Identity and Career Construction in Education* (pp. 58–77). IGI Global. doi:10.4018/978-1-5225-7772-0.ch004

Ashipala, D., Tomas, N., & Medusalem, J. M. (2020). Smoking. In S. G. Taukeni (Ed.), *Biopsychosocial Perspectives and Practices for Addressing Communicable and Non-Communicable Diseases* (pp. 85–104). IGI Global. doi:10.4018/978-1-7998-2139-7.ch006

Atiku, S. O. (2019). Institutionalizing Social Responsibility Through Workplace Green Behavior. In S. O. Atiku (Ed.), *Contemporary Multicultural Orientations and Practices for Global Leadership* (pp. 183–199). IGI Global. doi:10.4018/978-1-5225-6286-3.ch010

Aulet, S., & Tarrés, E. (2021). Tourism and Peacebuilding From a Holistic Approach. In Role and Impact of Tourism in Peacebuilding and Conflict Transformation (pp. 46-65). IGI Global. doi:10.4018/978-1-7998-5053-3.ch004

Baker, A., Iqbal, F., Laila, M., & Waheed, A. (2020). Psychology With Mahnoor App. In S. Umair (Ed.), *Mobile Devices and Smart Gadgets in Medical Sciences* (pp. 214–231). IGI Global. doi:10.4018/978-1-7998-2521-0.ch010

Baker, C., & Blankenship, R. J. (2019). Minority College Students and Digital Agency. In R. J. Blankenship (Ed.), *Critical Essays on the New Moral Imperative for Supporting Marginalized Students in PK-20 Education* (pp. 103–135). IGI Global. doi:10.4018/978-1-5225-7787-4.ch006

Balls-Berry, J. E., & Albold, C. (2019). Asynchronous Education for Graduate Medical Trainees to Reduce Health Disparities and Address Social Determinants of Health. In Optimizing Medical Education With Instructional Technology (pp. 1-20). IGI Global. doi:10.4018/978-1-5225-6289-4.ch001

Baragde, D. B., & Jadhav, A. U. (2020). Circular Economy Model for the E-Waste Management Sector. In N. Baporikar (Ed.), *Handbook of Research on Entrepreneurship Development and Opportunities in Circular Economy* (pp. 216–230). IGI Global. doi:10.4018/978-1-7998-5116-5.ch011

Battista, L. T., & Wright, L. (2020). Overcoming Implicit Bias in Collaborative Online Learning Communities. In C. N. Stevenson & J. C. Bauer (Eds.), *Enriching Collaboration and Communication in Online Learning Communities* (pp. 19–38). IGI Global. doi:10.4018/978-1-5225-9814-5.ch002

Baykal, E. (2019). Innovating Through Reflective Learning in Mindful Organizations. In H. Dinçer & S. Yüksel (Eds.), *Handbook of Research on Managerial Thinking in Global Business Economics* (pp. 246–261). IGI Global. doi:10.4018/978-1-5225-7180-3.ch014

Baykal, E. (2020). Mindfulness and Mindful Coaching. In E. Baykal (Ed.), *Handbook of Research on Positive Organizational Behavior for Improved Workplace Performance* (pp. 72–85). IGI Global. doi:10.4018/978-1-7998-0058-3.ch005

Bender, S., & Bratton, I. N. (2020). Housing Insecurities and Homelessness Among Children and Unaccompanied Youth in Rural Appalachian Communities. In H. C. Greene, B. S. Zugelder, & J. C. Manner (Eds.), *Handbook of Research on Leadership and Advocacy for Children and Families in Rural Poverty* (pp. 23–45). IGI Global. doi:10.4018/978-1-7998-2787-0.ch002

Benes, S. (2020). Health Education as a Tool for Social Justice and Health Equity. In S. T. Brand & L. E. Ciccomascolo (Eds.), *Social Justice and Putting Theory Into Practice in Schools and Communities* (pp. 58–80). IGI Global. doi:10.4018/978-1-5225-9434-5.ch005

Benvenuti, M., Błachnio, A., Przepiorka, A. M., Daskalova, V. M., & Mazzoni, E. (2020). Factors Related to Phone Snubbing Behavior in Emerging Adults. In M. Desjarlais (Ed.), *The Psychology and Dynamics Behind Social Media Interactions* (pp. 164–187). IGI Global. doi:10.4018/978-1-5225-9412-3.ch007

Benvenuti, M., Giovagnoli, S., Keep, M., Mazzoni, E., & Selleri, P. (2020). The Onlife in Emerging Adulthood. In M. F. Wright (Ed.), *Recent Advances in Digital Media Impacts on Identity, Sexuality, and Relationships* (pp. 241–264). IGI Global. doi:10.4018/978-1-7998-1063-6.ch013

Berkley-Patton, J., Thompson, C. B., Ervie, K. G., Huffman, M., & Johnson, N. R. (2020). Using a Community-Based Collaborative Care Model as a Platform for Successful Interprofessional Education. In Building a Patient-Centered Interprofessional Education Program (pp. 157-182). IGI Global. doi:10.4018/978-1-7998-3066-5.ch009

Bhattacharyya, S. S. (2019). Mergers and Acquisition by Indian Firms. In P. Ordoñez de Pablos (Ed.), *Dynamic Perspectives on Globalization and Sustainable Business in Asia* (pp. 41–55). IGI Global. doi:10.4018/978-1-5225-7095-0.ch004

Bianchi, S. (2019). Spirituality in the Workplace. In D. Mishra (Ed.), *Science and Spirituality for a Sustainable World* (pp. 153–174). IGI Global. doi:10.4018/978-1-5225-9893-0.ch009

Bilmez, B., & Aral, N. (2020). Yoga for Babies and Children. In N. Aral (Ed.), *Handbook of Research on Prenatal, Postnatal, and Early Childhood Development* (pp. 386–397). IGI Global. doi:10.4018/978-1-7998-2952-2.ch021

Bisen, S. S., & Deshpande, Y. (2019). The Repercussion of the Internet on Psychological Wellbeing. In B. Bozoglan (Ed.), *Multifaceted Approach to Digital Addiction and Its Treatment* (pp. 101–117). IGI Global. doi:10.4018/978-1-5225-8449-0.ch005

Bishop, J. (2018). Evaluating the Risk of Digital Addiction in Blended Learning Environments: Considering ICT Intensity, Learning Style, and Architecture. In B. Bozoglan (Ed.), *Psychological, Social, and Cultural Aspects of Internet Addiction* (pp. 169–185). IGI Global. doi:10.4018/978-1-5225-3477-8.ch009

Bishop, J. (2019). Conceptualizing Digital Addiction as Glutamine Inhibition and Glutamate Acceleration (GIGA). In B. Bozoglan (Ed.), *Multifaceted Approach to Digital Addiction and Its Treatment* (pp. 73–99). IGI Global. doi:10.4018/978-1-5225-8449-0.ch004

Bishop, J. (2019). Quantifying Participation in Large-Scale Virtual Environments. In B. Bozoglan (Ed.), *Multifaceted Approach to Digital Addiction and Its Treatment* (pp. 177–206). IGI Global. doi:10.4018/978-1-5225-8449-0.ch009

Blomeley, S., & Hamilton, A. H. (2018). Writing Partners. In O. O. Delano-Oriaran, M. W. Penick-Parks, & S. Fondrie (Eds.), *Culturally Engaging Service-Learning With Diverse Communities* (pp. 202–222). IGI Global. doi:10.4018/978-1-5225-2900-2.ch012

Bopp, J. (2019). Storytelling Through Dance and Movement. In J. Bopp, A. M. Grebe, & J. H. Denny (Eds.), *Healing Through the Arts for Non-Clinical Practitioners* (pp. 124–155). IGI Global. doi:10.4018/978-1-5225-5981-8.ch009

Boursier, V., & Manna, V. (2019). Relational Body Identities. In R. T. Gopalan (Ed.), *Intimacy and Developing Personal Relationships in the Virtual World* (pp. 40–63). IGI Global. doi:10.4018/978-1-5225-4047-2.ch003

Bozoglan, B. (2018). The Role of Family Factors in Internet Addiction Among Children and Adolescents. In B. Bozoglan (Ed.), *Psychological, Social, and Cultural Aspects of Internet Addiction* (pp. 146–168). IGI Global. doi:10.4018/978-1-5225-3477-8.ch008

Bozoglan, B. (2019). Systemic Approach and Digital Addiction. In B. Bozoglan (Ed.), *Multifaceted Approach to Digital Addiction and Its Treatment* (pp. 260–280). IGI Global. doi:10.4018/978-1-5225-8449-0.ch012

Bozoglan, B. (2019). The Impact of Family on Digital Addiction. In B. Bozoglan (Ed.), *Multifaceted Approach to Digital Addiction and Its Treatment* (pp. 20–45). IGI Global. doi:10.4018/978-1-5225-8449-0.ch002

Bresciani Ludvik, M. (2020). A New Era of Accountability. In Higher Education Response to Exponential Societal Shifts (pp. 251-274). IGI Global. http:// doi:10.4018/978-1-7998-2410-7.ch012

Brewer, O., & Erdem, O. (2020). Values Activation and Present Bias. *International Journal of Applied Behavioral Economics*, *9*(2), 57–69. doi:10.4018/IJABE.2020040104

Brkljačić, T., Sučić, I., Tkalić, R. G., Wertag, A., & Lučić, L. (2019). Games We Play. In B. Bozoglan (Ed.), *Multifaceted Approach to Digital Addiction and Its Treatment* (pp. 118–137). IGI Global. doi:10.4018/978-1-5225-8449-0.ch006

Brooks, S., Wang, X., & Schneider, C. (2020). Technology Addictions and Technostress. *Journal of Organizational and End User Computing*, *32*(2), 1–19. doi:10.4018/JOEUC.2020040101

Brussier, I. C. (2020). Conduct Disorder and Oppositional Defiant Disorder. In N. R. Silton (Ed.), *Exploring Best Child Development Practices in Contemporary Society* (pp. 166–190). IGI Global. doi:10.4018/978-1-7998-2940-9.ch008

Burrell, D. N., Shufutinsky, A., Bland, S., Cole, C. M., Wright, J. B., Crowe, M., Aridi, A. S., & Mairs-Levy, J. (2020). A Case Study of a Hospital Workplace Culture of Injustice for Women Physicians. *International Journal of Patient-Centered Healthcare*, *10*(1), 15–36. doi:10.4018/IJPCH.2020010102

Celosse, K. (2018). Interactions Between Personality Traits of Law Enforcement and Corrections Officers, and Attitudes Toward Felony Drug Offenders. In F. S. Topor (Ed.), *Ethical Standards and Practice in International Relations* (pp. 128–156). IGI Global. doi:10.4018/978-1-5225-2650-6.ch006

Cesari, S. (2020). Prison Treatment Programs From an International Perspective. In A. Balloni & R. Sette (Eds.), *Handbook of Research on Trends and Issues in Crime Prevention, Rehabilitation, and Victim Support* (pp. 359–374). IGI Global. doi:10.4018/978-1-7998-1286-9.ch021

Cherner, T. S., & Kokopeli, E. M. (2018). Using Web 2.0 Tools to Start a WebQuest Renaissance. In A. A. Khan & S. Umair (Eds.), *Handbook of Research on Mobile Devices and Smart Gadgets in K-12 Education* (pp. 134–148). IGI Global. doi:10.4018/978-1-5225-2706-0.ch010

Choi, Y. (2020). A Study of the Influence of Social Media Use on Employees' Psychological Distress and the Moderating Effect of Perceived Organizational Support. *International Journal of Human Capital and Information Technology Professionals*, *11*(3), 23–36. doi:10.4018/IJHCITP.2020070102

Choi, Y. (2020). Corporate Psychopathy and Internet Video Game Addiction in the Workplace. *International Journal of Gaming and Computer-Mediated Simulations*, *12*(3), 18–36. doi:10.4018/IJGCMS.2020070102

Choudhury, S. (2021). ADHD in Children. In R. T. Gopalan (Ed.), *New Developments in Diagnosing, Assessing, and Treating ADHD* (pp. 55–69). IGI Global. doi:10.4018/978-1-7998-5495-1.ch004

Cline, B. J. (2020). Assessment and Civility. In C. N. Stevenson & J. C. Bauer (Eds.), *Enriching Collaboration and Communication in Online Learning Communities* (pp. 39–51). IGI Global. doi:10.4018/978-1-5225-9814-5.ch003

Daniel, A. (2019). An Integral View of Mindfulness Practices and the Perception of Challenge Within a High School Setting. In V. Bohac Clarke (Ed.), *Integral Theory and Transdisciplinary Action Research in Education* (pp. 182–207). IGI Global. doi:10.4018/978-1-5225-5873-6.ch009

Dard, D. (2019). Unlocking the Gate to Inner Peace With Yoga. In M. W. Lutfy & C. Toffolo (Eds.), *Handbook of Research on Promoting Peace Through Practice, Academia, and the Arts* (pp. 147–164). IGI Global. doi:10.4018/978-1-5225-3001-5.ch008

De Giuseppe, T., & Corona, F. (2020). Flipped Inclusion Between Educational Emergencies and Transformative Socio-Semiotic Didactics. In *Disruptive and Emerging Technology Trends Across Education and the Workplace* (pp. 52-89). IGI Global. http://doi:10.4018/978-1-7998-2914-0.ch003

Delello, J. A., Kiekel, J., Poyo, S. R., Williams, M. K., & Kerby, D. (2020). Educator Perceptions of Digital Devices. In J. A. Delello & R. R. McWhorter (Eds.), *Disruptive and Emerging Technology Trends Across Education and the Workplace* (pp. 193–220). IGI Global. doi:10.4018/978-1-7998-2914-0.ch008

Demirtepe-Saygili, D. (2020). Stress, Coping, and Social Media Use. In M. Desjarlais (Ed.), *The Psychology and Dynamics Behind Social Media Interactions* (pp. 241–267). IGI Global. doi:10.4018/978-1-5225-9412-3.ch010

Donmez, B., & Seneler, C. (2019). Locating Gender Differences in Mobile Use and Habits. In X. Xu (Ed.), *Impacts of Mobile Use and Experience on Contemporary Society* (pp. 37–52). IGI Global. doi:10.4018/978-1-5225-7885-7.ch003

Downey, L. L., & Cohen, M. S. (2018). Virtual Worlds and Well-Being. *International Journal of Virtual and Augmented Reality, 2*(1), 14–31. doi:10.4018/IJVAR.2018010102

Duckworth, G., & Krouse, A. (2020). Look Up. In J. A. Delello & R. R. McWhorter (Eds.), *Disruptive and Emerging Technology Trends Across Education and the Workplace* (pp. 269–293). IGI Global. doi:10.4018/978-1-7998-2914-0.ch011

Eisenhauer, M. J., Gregory, A. E., & Cahill, M. A. (2020). Stemming the Opioid Crisis With Three-Year-Olds in Rural America. In H. C. Greene, B. S. Zugelder, & J. C. Manner (Eds.), *Handbook of Research on Leadership and Advocacy for Children and Families in Rural Poverty* (pp. 75–97). IGI Global. doi:10.4018/978-1-7998-2787-0.ch004

Ekenene, G. E. (2020). Culture of Safety and Good Health. In E. Essien (Ed.), *Handbook of Research on the Impact of Culture in Conflict Prevention and Peacebuilding* (pp. 154–175). IGI Global. doi:10.4018/978-1-7998-2574-6.ch010

Elliott, L. J. (2020). The Impact of User Experience With Technology on Course Expectations. In Handbook of Research on Adult Learning in Higher Education (pp. 598-632). IGI Global. doi:10.4018/978-1-7998-1306-4.ch023

Elrashedy, A. A. (2018). HIV-Associated Neurocognitive Disorder. In A. Al Mazari (Ed.), *Big Data Analytics in HIV/AIDS Research* (pp. 171–205). IGI Global. doi:10.4018/978-1-5225-3203-3.ch008

Erben, G. S. (2019). Mindfulness as an Antecedent of Work Engagement. In N. Sharma, N. Chaudhary, & V. K. Singh (Eds.), *Management Techniques for Employee Engagement in Contemporary Organizations* (pp. 126–141). IGI Global. doi:10.4018/978-1-5225-7799-7.ch008

Erden, N. S. (2019). Do Organizations Really Gain Without Pain? In N. Sharma, N. Chaudhary, & V. K. Singh (Eds.), *Management Techniques for Employee Engagement in Contemporary Organizations* (pp. 57–76). IGI Global. doi:10.4018/978-1-5225-7799-7.ch004

Evans, G., Hamerston, L., Cherrett, L. M., & Sadd, D. J. (2018). The Use of Systems Thinking, Systems Practice, to Elicit the Effectiveness of Cancer Support Services in the Southwest of England. *International Journal of Systems and Society, 5*(2), 13–29. doi:10.4018/IJSS.2018070102

Evans, S. F., & Howarth, M. (2019). I Am Happy, So I Learn It. In P. D. Keough (Ed.), *Ethical Problem-Solving and Decision-Making for Positive and Conclusive Outcomes* (pp. 101–122). IGI Global. doi:10.4018/978-1-5225-7582-5.ch006

Ezoe, S., Iida, T., Inoue, K., & Toda, M. (2019). Smartphone Addiction and Sleep Quality Associated with Depression in University Students in Japan. *International Journal of Cyber Behavior, Psychology and Learning*, *9*(4), 22–31. doi:10.4018/IJCBPL.2019100102

Ezoe, S., & Toda, M. (2019). Relationships of Smartphone Dependence With Chronotype and Gender in Adolescence. In Z. Yan (Ed.), *Analyzing Human Behavior in Cyberspace* (pp. 39–59). IGI Global. doi:10.4018/978-1-5225-7128-5.ch003

Flynn, C. F. (2020). Facilitating Civility in Distance Education. In K. Setzekorn, N. Patnayakuni, & T. Burton (Eds.), *Socioeconomics, Diversity, and the Politics of Online Education* (pp. 1–16). IGI Global. doi:10.4018/978-1-7998-3583-7.ch001

Gallego, J. (2020). Cultivating Cultural Self-Awareness. In R. Brunet-Thornton (Ed.), *Examining Cultural Perspectives in a Globalized World* (pp. 65–93). IGI Global. doi:10.4018/978-1-7998-0214-3.ch004

Gao, T., & Wang, G. Y. (2020). Brain Signal Classification Based on Deep CNN. *International Journal of Security and Privacy in Pervasive Computing*, *12*(2), 17–29. doi:10.4018/IJSPPC.2020040102

Gardner, N. S., Luke, K. J., Wheatley, A. O., De La Haye, W., Bahado-Singh, P. S., Dilworth, L. L., McGrowder, D. A., Barton, E., Young-Martin, L. E., Salako-Akande, A., Lowe, H., Morrison, E., Eldermire-Shearer, D., & Asemota, H. (2019). Plasma Cocaine Metabolite Levels and Liver CYP450 3A4 Isoenzyme Activity as Indicators of Cocaine Metabolism in Rats Treated With Salako Supplements. In S. Palchoudhury (Ed.), *Strategic Applications of Measurement Technologies and Instrumentation* (pp. 1–21). IGI Global. doi:10.4018/978-1-5225-5406-6.ch001

Gautam, S., & Dada, R. (2021). Molecular Mechanisms Underlying the Effects of Yoga. In S. Telles & R. K. Gupta (Eds.), *Handbook of Research on Evidence-Based Perspectives on the Psychophysiology of Yoga and Its Applications* (pp. 103–123). IGI Global. doi:10.4018/978-1-7998-3254-6.ch007

Gauthier-Pin, S. (2019). The Magic of Monologue. In J. Bopp, A. M. Grebe, & J. H. Denny (Eds.), *Healing Through the Arts for Non-Clinical Practitioners* (pp. 75–85). IGI Global. doi:10.4018/978-1-5225-5981-8.ch006

Gavurova, B., & Kubak, M. (2021). Distribution of Selected Health Technology in Regions of Slovakia. In Encyclopedia of Information Science and Technology, Fifth Edition (pp. 1872-1886). IGI Global. doi:10.4018/978-1-7998-3479-3.ch130

Gilchrist-Petty, E. (2018). *Student Resistance*. IGI Global. doi:10.4018/978-1-5225-2779-4.ch002

Gioia, F., & Boursier, V. (2019). Treatment of Internet Addiction and Internet Gaming Disorder in Adolescence. In B. Bozoglan (Ed.), *Multifaceted Approach to Digital Addiction and Its Treatment* (pp. 157–176). IGI Global. doi:10.4018/978-1-5225-8449-0.ch008

Gomez, B. J., & Ang, P. M. (2021). Emotional Intelligence 4.0. In M. R. Gurubatham & G. A. Williams (Eds.), *Advancing Innovation and Sustainable Outcomes in International Graduate Education* (pp. 53–68). IGI Global. doi:10.4018/978-1-7998-5514-9.ch004

Gopalan, R. T. (2021). ADHD Symptoms, Comorbidities, Social, and Familial Adversities on Offences. In R. T. Gopalan (Ed.), *New Developments in Diagnosing, Assessing, and Treating ADHD* (pp. 259–277). IGI Global. doi:10.4018/978-1-7998-5495-1.ch017

Gopalan, R. T. (2021). ADHD, Parental Stress, Stigma, and Mindfulness Training. In R. T. Gopalan (Ed.), *New Developments in Diagnosing, Assessing, and Treating ADHD* (pp. 278–304). IGI Global. doi:10.4018/978-1-7998-5495-1.ch018

Goyal, S., & Bhalla, P. (2020). A Review Study of the Effects of Personality Traits on Destructive and Constructive Deviance. In N. Sharma (Ed.), *Analyzing Workplace Deviance in Modern Organizations* (pp. 187–202). IGI Global. doi:10.4018/978-1-5225-9996-8.ch010

Guest, J. D., & Williams-Thompson, K. (2021). Addressing the Parallel Process, Countertransference, and Resistance in Supervision Using Play and Expressive Arts Techniques. In L. J. Fazio-Griffith & R. Marino (Eds.), *Techniques and Interventions for Play Therapy and Clinical Supervision* (pp. 84–105). IGI Global. doi:10.4018/978-1-7998-4628-4.ch006

Güvenç Salabğir, Z., & Nasır, S. (2020). Investigation of Smartphone Use Addiction in Generation Y. In M. F. Wright (Ed.), *Recent Advances in Digital Media Impacts on Identity, Sexuality, and Relationships* (pp. 190–205). IGI Global. doi:10.4018/978-1-7998-1063-6.ch010

Hai-Jew, S. (2020). Recognizing Curricular Infusions in Extant Online Learning Contents by Types and at Varying Scales. In S. Hai-Jew (Ed.), *Form, Function, and Style in Instructional Design* (pp. 105–133). IGI Global. doi:10.4018/978-1-5225-9833-6.ch006

Hampton-Garland, P., Sechrest-Ehrhardt, L., & Cooke, B. (2018). *S.N.A.P. Today, Medicare Tomorrow*. IGI Global. doi:10.4018/978-1-5225-3843-1.ch004

Hamutoğlu, N. B., Topal, M., Samur, Y., Gezgin, D. M., & Griffiths, M. D. (2020). The Development of the Online Player Type Scale. *International Journal of Cyber Behavior, Psychology and Learning*, *10*(1), 15–31. doi:10.4018/IJCBPL.2020010102

Hartley, M. L. (2020). Mind, Brain, and Education. In H. C. Greene, B. S. Zugelder, & J. C. Manner (Eds.), *Handbook of Research on Leadership and Advocacy for Children and Families in Rural Poverty* (pp. 259–278). IGI Global. doi:10.4018/978-1-7998-2787-0.ch012

Heasley, T. (2020). Addressing the Need for Anger Management in Young People. In S. G. Taukeni (Ed.), *Addressing Multicultural Needs in School Guidance and Counseling* (pp. 33–63). IGI Global. doi:10.4018/978-1-7998-0319-5.ch003

Hege, A., Presnell, D., Reed-Ashcraft, K. B., Caldwell, K., Pyles, D. G., Bouldin, E. D., & Warren, J. (2020). Advocacy and Action in Appalachia Aimed at Adverse Childhood Experiences. In H. C. Greene, B. S. Zugelder, & J. C. Manner (Eds.), *Handbook of Research on Leadership and Advocacy for Children and Families in Rural Poverty* (pp. 125–148). IGI Global. doi:10.4018/978-1-7998-2787-0.ch006

Ifijeh, G., Ilogho, J., Iwu-James, J., Michael-Onuoha, H. C., & Osinulu, I. (2019). Social Media Use in Academic Libraries. In J. Joe & E. Knight (Eds.), *Social Media for Communication and Instruction in Academic Libraries* (pp. 237–257). IGI Global. doi:10.4018/978-1-5225-8097-3.ch014

Ignacimuthu, L., & Kumar, M. V. (2020). Theories of Social Media and Learning. In Innovations and Technologies for Soft Skill Development and Learning (pp. 142-154). IGI Global. http://doi:10.4018/978-1-7998-3464-9.ch017

Ilter, A., & Karacar, P. (2020). Mobile Technology and Social Media Literacy. In N. O. Taskiran (Ed.), *Handbook of Research on Multidisciplinary Approaches to Literacy in the Digital Age* (pp. 180–196). IGI Global. doi:10.4018/978-1-7998-1534-1.ch010

Isah, A., & Ogundele, O. R. (2020). Exploring the Use of Social Media as Tools for Information Sharing Among Undergraduates of University of Ilorin. In A. Tella (Ed.), *Handbook of Research on Digital Devices for Inclusivity and Engagement in Libraries* (pp. 297–306). IGI Global. doi:10.4018/978-1-5225-9034-7.ch015

Islam, M. A., & Kumar, B. (2020). Nexus Between Social Network, Social Media Use, and Loneliness. In P. Ordoñez de Pablos, X. Zhang, & K. Chui (Eds.), *Innovative Management and Business Practices in Asia* (pp. 228–243). IGI Global. doi:10.4018/978-1-7998-1566-2.ch012

Jain, S., Alam, M. A., & Kazmi, N. A. (2020). Psychological Impact and Assessment of Youth for the Use of Social Network. In E. C. Idemudia (Ed.), *Handbook of Research on Social and Organizational Dynamics in the Digital Era* (pp. 344–382). IGI Global. doi:10.4018/978-1-5225-8933-4.ch017

Jain, S., & Raju, S. (2018). Subjective Fatigue in Children and Adults. In S. K. Gupta & S. Venkatesan (Eds.), *Handbook of Research on Psychosocial Perspectives of Human Communication Disorders* (pp. 184–208). IGI Global. doi:10.4018/978-1-5225-4955-0.ch010

Jarvis, P. (2018). Deconstructing the Social Network. In I. Tshabangu (Ed.), *Global Ideologies Surrounding Children's Rights and Social Justice* (pp. 106–127). IGI Global. doi:10.4018/978-1-5225-2578-3.ch007

Jean-Baptiste, A. M., & Asongwed, E. T. (2018). Service Learning as an Approach to Combatting the Triad of Interrelated Diseases in the District of Columbia. In Changing Urban Landscapes Through Public Higher Education (pp. 26-56). IGI Global. doi:10.4018/978-1-5225-3454-9.ch002

Johns, E. (2020). Lucille. In B. C. King & T. A. Stewart (Eds.), *Cases on Cross-Cultural Counseling Strategies* (pp. 305–325). IGI Global. doi:10.4018/978-1-7998-0022-4.ch015

Johnson, L. W. (2020). Healthcare Considerations for the Hispanic Population. In D. M. Scott (Ed.), *Cases on Communication Disorders in Culturally Diverse Populations* (pp. 239–259). IGI Global. doi:10.4018/978-1-7998-2261-5.ch012

Johnson, L. W. (2020). Traumatic Brain Injury in Culturally Diverse Populations. In D. M. Scott (Ed.), *Cases on Communication Disorders in Culturally Diverse Populations* (pp. 260–279). IGI Global. doi:10.4018/978-1-7998-2261-5.ch013

Joshi, H., & Mentor, D. (2018). Conceptualizing Experiential Learning for Computer-Mediated Engagement. In D. Mentor (Ed.), *Computer-Mediated Learning for Workforce Development* (pp. 251–271). IGI Global. doi:10.4018/978-1-5225-4111-0.ch013

Karani, A. M., & Achuthan, S. (2019). Classroom Behavior Among Management Students in the Higher Education of India. In S. R. Nair & J. Saiz-Álvarez (Eds.), *Handbook of Research on Ethics, Entrepreneurship, and Governance in Higher Education* (pp. 26–53). IGI Global. doi:10.4018/978-1-5225-5837-8.ch002

Kaushik, P. (2018). Promoting Successful Positive Aging Across the Health Continuum. In B. V. Prasad & S. Akbar (Eds.), *Handbook of Research on Geriatric Health, Treatment, and Care* (pp. 48–67). IGI Global. doi:10.4018/978-1-5225-3480-8.ch003

Kieu, T. A., & Le, T. D. (2020). Mindfulness Approach to Ethical Consumption. In B. R. Hernández-Sánchez, J. C. Sánchez-García, & A. C. Moreira (Eds.), *Building an Entrepreneurial and Sustainable Society* (pp. 289–304). IGI Global. doi:10.4018/978-1-7998-2704-7.ch015

Kiran, T., & Sharma, A. (2020). Role of Gender in Counterproductive Work Behavior. In N. Sharma (Ed.), *Analyzing Workplace Deviance in Modern Organizations* (pp. 79–99). IGI Global. doi:10.4018/978-1-5225-9996-8.ch005

Kirsch, B. (2020). Virtual Reality in Libraries. In B. Holland (Ed.), *Emerging Trends and Impacts of the Internet of Things in Libraries* (pp. 180–193). IGI Global. doi:10.4018/978-1-7998-4742-7.ch010

Knepper, H. (2018). Healthcare in the United States. In H. Levine & K. Moreno (Eds.), *Positioning Markets and Governments in Public Management* (pp. 73–85). IGI Global. doi:10.4018/978-1-5225-4177-6.ch007

Koç, T., & Akbıyık, A. (2020). Social Network Sites (SNS) and Their Irrepressible Popularity. In S. Alavi & V. Ahuja (Eds.), *Managing Social Media Practices in the Digital Economy* (pp. 234–263). IGI Global. doi:10.4018/978-1-7998-2185-4.ch011

Konecny, L. T. (2018). Medical School Wellness Initiatives. In C. R. Smith (Ed.), *Exploring the Pressures of Medical Education From a Mental Health and Wellness Perspective* (pp. 209–228). IGI Global. doi:10.4018/978-1-5225-2811-1.ch009

Kovacs, R. S. (2019). The Philip Seymour Hoffman Project. In M. N. Yildiz, M. Fazal, M. Ahn, R. Feirsen, & S. Ozdemir (Eds.), *Handbook of Research on Media Literacy Research and Applications Across Disciplines* (pp. 335–350). IGI Global. doi:10.4018/978-1-5225-9261-7.ch020

Krishnamurthy, K., & Ponnuswamy, M. J. (2018). Coupling of Optimization Algorithms Based on Swarm Intelligence. In U. Kose, G. E. Guraksin, & O. Deperlioglu (Eds.), *Nature-Inspired Intelligent Techniques for Solving Biomedical Engineering Problems* (pp. 27–50). IGI Global. doi:10.4018/978-1-5225-4769-3.ch002

Kumar, P., & Singh, G. (2020). Using Social Media and Digital Marketing Tools and Techniques for Developing Brand Equity With Connected Consumers. In S. S. Dadwal (Ed.), *Handbook of Research on Innovations in Technology and Marketing for the Connected Consumer* (pp. 336–355). IGI Global. doi:10.4018/978-1-7998-0131-3.ch016

Kumara, C. N. (2019). Religion in Therapy. In A. J. Jegathesan & S. S. Abdullah (Eds.), *Multicultural Counseling Applications for Improved Mental Healthcare Services* (pp. 235–250). IGI Global. doi:10.4018/978-1-5225-6073-9.ch015

Lafer, E. M., McCuiston, M., & Swanson, A. (2021). Yoga Therapy. In S. Telles & R. K. Gupta (Eds.), *Handbook of Research on Evidence-Based Perspectives on the Psychophysiology of Yoga and Its Applications* (pp. 159–178). IGI Global. doi:10.4018/978-1-7998-3254-6.ch010

Lai, F. T., & Kwan, J. L. (2018). Socioeconomic Determinants of Internet Addiction in Adolescents. In B. Bozoglan (Ed.), *Psychological, Social, and Cultural Aspects of Internet Addiction* (pp. 127–145). IGI Global. doi:10.4018/978-1-5225-3477-8.ch007

Lane, H., Martin, J. M., & Haines, T. (2019). Healthcare Decision Making. In J. M. Martin (Ed.), *Mental Health Policy, Practice, and Service Accessibility in Contemporary Society* (pp. 41–56). IGI Global. doi:10.4018/978-1-5225-7402-6.ch003

Larsen, T. (2019). Neuroeconomic Psychology. *International Journal of Patient-Centered Healthcare*, *9*(1), 1–17. doi:10.4018/IJPCH.2019010101

Lewis, A. S. (2019). What's Respect Got to Do With It? In U. Thomas (Ed.), *Navigating Micro-Aggressions Toward Women in Higher Education* (pp. 181–201). IGI Global. doi:10.4018/978-1-5225-5942-9.ch009

Lilly, M. M., Dadouch, Z., & Robinson, D. A. (2020). The First, First Responder. In Mental Health Intervention and Treatment of First Responders and Emergency Workers (pp. 63-85). IGI Global. http://doi:10.4018/978-1-5225-9803-9.ch005

Loehr, G. T., Shackleford, L., Dill-Shackleford, K. E., & Metcalf, M. (2020). Sci-Fi Fandoms in the Digital Age. In C. L. Wang (Ed.), *Handbook of Research on the Impact of Fandom in Society and Consumerism* (pp. 305–322). IGI Global. doi:10.4018/978-1-7998-1048-3.ch015

Mackinem, M. B., & Sporl, C. (2020). A Primer on Substance Use and Islam. In A. Bagasra & M. Mackinem (Eds.), *Working With Muslim Clients in the Helping Professions* (pp. 23–39). IGI Global. doi:10.4018/978-1-7998-0018-7.ch002

Maiti, T. (2019). Internet Addiction and Online Gaming. In R. T. Gopalan (Ed.), *Intimacy and Developing Personal Relationships in the Virtual World* (pp. 174–200). IGI Global. doi:10.4018/978-1-5225-4047-2.ch010

Maiti, T., & Hasija, A. D. (2021). ADHD and Addiction. In R. T. Gopalan (Ed.), *New Developments in Diagnosing, Assessing, and Treating ADHD* (pp. 229–244). IGI Global. doi:10.4018/978-1-7998-5495-1.ch015

Manuel, J. J. (2021). Special Yoga for Children and Young People With Special Needs. In S. Telles & R. K. Gupta (Eds.), *Handbook of Research on Evidence-Based Perspectives on the Psychophysiology of Yoga and Its Applications* (pp. 330–346). IGI Global. doi:10.4018/978-1-7998-3254-6.ch019

Martin, M., Mockry, J., Puliatte, A., Simard, D., & Squires, M. (2018). *Strategies for the College Classroom*. IGI Global. doi:10.4018/978-1-5225-3793-9.ch004

Mattoo, S. K., Punia, V., Malik, L., & Khurana, H. (2018). Spirituality and Aging. In B. V. Prasad & S. Akbar (Eds.), *Handbook of Research on Geriatric Health, Treatment, and Care* (pp. 17–47). IGI Global. doi:10.4018/978-1-5225-3480-8.ch002

Mayo, S. (2018). A Collective Consciousness Model in a Post-Media Society. In Enhancing Art, Culture, and Design With Technological Integration (pp. 25-49). IGI Global. doi:10.4018/978-1-5225-5023-5.ch002

McKain, D. (2019). Adolescent Chronic Stress. In A. Starcevic (Ed.), *Chronic Stress and Its Effect on Brain Structure and Connectivity* (pp. 46–72). IGI Global. doi:10.4018/978-1-5225-7513-9.ch002

McKain, D. (2019). Outdoor Approaches for Smartphone Addiction. In B. Bozoglan (Ed.), *Multifaceted Approach to Digital Addiction and Its Treatment* (pp. 292–308). IGI Global. doi:10.4018/978-1-5225-8449-0.ch014

McKain, D., & Grise, J. B. (2019). Finding Balance. In H. L. Schnackenberg & C. Johnson (Eds.), *Preparing the Higher Education Space for Gen Z* (pp. 1–31). IGI Global. doi:10.4018/978-1-5225-7763-8.ch001

Messer, D., Shanholtz, C. E., & Chowdhury, A. (2019). Digital Behavior Change Interventions. In Z. Yan (Ed.), *Analyzing Human Behavior in Cyberspace* (pp. 124–138). IGI Global. doi:10.4018/978-1-5225-7128-5.ch008

Miltenoff, P., & Milne, K. (2020). Educators and Wellbeing. In S. P. Huffman, S. Loyless, S. Albritton, & C. Green (Eds.), *Leveraging Technology to Improve School Safety and Student Wellbeing* (pp. 86–101). IGI Global. doi:10.4018/978-1-7998-1766-6.ch006

Misra, R., Singh, S., & Singh, N. (2020). Assessing Behavioral Patterns for Online Gaming Addiction. *International Journal of Cyber Behavior, Psychology and Learning*, *10*(2), 43–64. doi:10.4018/IJCBPL.2020040104

Mocenni, C., Montefrancesco, G., & Tiezzi, S. (2019). A Model of Spontaneous Remission From Addiction. *International Journal of Applied Behavioral Economics*, *8*(1), 21–48. doi:10.4018/IJABE.2019010102

Moerman, J., Braaksma, J., & van Dongen, L. A. (2019). Assessing HRO Principles for Reliable Performance in Asset-Intensive Organizations. In V. G. Diaz & J. Bonilla (Eds.), *Handbook of Research on Industrial Advancement in Scientific Knowledge* (pp. 160–181). IGI Global. doi:10.4018/978-1-5225-7152-0.ch009

Mohan, A., & Ravindran, S. K. (2020). Loneliness and Problematic Internet Use Among Young Adults. *International Journal of Cyber Behavior, Psychology and Learning*, *10*(2), 19–30. doi:10.4018/IJCBPL.2020040102

Mohan, G. (2021). Traditional Frameworks of Well-Being and Modern Science. In S. Telles & R. K. Gupta (Eds.), *Handbook of Research on Evidence-Based Perspectives on the Psychophysiology of Yoga and Its Applications* (pp. 410–421). IGI Global. doi:10.4018/978-1-7998-3254-6.ch023

Morningstar, J., & Dibb, J. (2021). The Science and Art of Contemporary Breathwork and Yoga. In Handbook of Research on Evidence-Based Perspectives on the Psychophysiology of Yoga and Its Applications (pp. 422-450). IGI Global. http://doi:10.4018/978-1-7998-3254-6.ch024

Mukonza, C., & Swarts, I. (2019). Examining the Role of Green Transformational Leadership on Promoting Green Organizational Behavior. In S. O. Atiku (Ed.), *Contemporary Multicultural Orientations and Practices for Global Leadership* (pp. 200–224). IGI Global. doi:10.4018/978-1-5225-6286-3.ch011

Murdoch, R. (2019). Serious Games, Meditation, Brain-Computer Interfacing, and Virtual Reality (VR). In G. Guazzaroni (Ed.), *Virtual and Augmented Reality in Mental Health Treatment* (pp. 32–50). IGI Global. doi:10.4018/978-1-5225-7168-1.ch003

Nagarajah, J., Mejer, J. S., & See, N. L. (2020). Life Skills in University Curricula. In P. Kumar, M. J. Keppell, & C. L. Lim (Eds.), *Preparing 21st Century Teachers for Teach Less, Learn More (TLLM) Pedagogies* (pp. 82–106). IGI Global. doi:10.4018/978-1-7998-1435-1.ch006

Nagpal, A. (2019). Understanding the Psychology of New Media Audiences From a Marketing Perspective. In P. Mishra & S. O. Dham (Eds.), *Application of Gaming in New Media Marketing* (pp. 112–124). IGI Global. doi:10.4018/978-1-5225-6064-7.ch007

Narang, R., & Tiwari, S. (2021). Antecedents and Consequences of the Growing Popularity of Digital Consumption. In Encyclopedia of Information Science and Technology, Fifth Edition (pp. 1066-1084). IGI Global. doi:10.4018/978-1-7998-3479-3.ch073

Nyamadi, M. (2020). Technology Addictions, Model Development, Measurement, and Effect on Performance From a Developing Country Context. In R. Boateng (Ed.), *Handbook of Research on Managing Information Systems in Developing Economies* (pp. 471–479). IGI Global. doi:10.4018/978-1-7998-2610-1.ch023

O'Brien, T. (2019). Bringing Cross-Cultural Communication Analysis Into Foreign Language Classrooms. In P. Romanowski & E. Bandura (Eds.), *Intercultural Foreign Language Teaching and Learning in Higher Education Contexts* (pp. 71–97). IGI Global. doi:10.4018/978-1-5225-8128-4.ch004

O'Donnell, E., & O'Donnell, L. (2020). The Dark Side of Engaging With Social Networking Sites (SNS). In Encyclopedia of Criminal Activities and the Deep Web (pp. 615-627). IGI Global. http://doi:10.4018/978-1-5225-9715-5.ch042

Ogundoyin, O. S. (2020). Role of the Media on Migrants' Vulnerability to Health Hazards. In N. Okorie, B. R. Ojebuyi, & J. W. Macharia (Eds.), *Handbook of Research on the Global Impact of Media on Migration Issues* (pp. 142–156). IGI Global. doi:10.4018/978-1-7998-0210-5.ch009

Oh, S. K., Hong, S., & Park, H. S. (2020). The Tipping Point. *International Journal of Social Media and Online Communities*, *12*(1), 23–39. doi:10.4018/IJSMOC.2020010103

Ok, C. (2020). How Growing Older Leads to Different Patterns in Smartphone Usage Among Genders. *International Journal of Mobile Human Computer Interaction*, *12*(3), 46–59. doi:10.4018/IJMHCI.2020070103

Olsen, E. H. (2021). Yoga as a Healing Modality of Trauma-Related Symptoms and Disorders. In S. Telles & R. K. Gupta (Eds.), *Handbook of Research on Evidence-Based Perspectives on the Psychophysiology of Yoga and Its Applications* (pp. 199–220). IGI Global. doi:10.4018/978-1-7998-3254-6.ch012

Olson-Morrison, D. L. (2021). Virtual Reality in Social Work Education. In D. H. Choi, A. Dailey-Hebert, & J. S. Estes (Eds.), *Current and Prospective Applications of Virtual Reality in Higher Education* (pp. 232–256). IGI Global. doi:10.4018/978-1-7998-4960-5.ch011

Olszewski, C. A., & Hansman, C. A. (2020). Faculty Socialization and Gaining Tenure. In V. Wang (Ed.), *Handbook of Research on Ethical Challenges in Higher Education Leadership and Administration* (pp. 51–71). IGI Global. doi:10.4018/978-1-7998-4141-8.ch004

Omoruyi, E. A., & Omidele, F. (2018). Resident Physician and Medical Academic Faculty Burnout. In C. R. Smith (Ed.), *Exploring the Pressures of Medical Education From a Mental Health and Wellness Perspective* (pp. 171–189). IGI Global. doi:10.4018/978-1-5225-2811-1.ch007

Opengart, R., Reio, T. G. Jr, & Ding, W. (2019). Workplace Incivility and Job Satisfaction. *International Journal of Adult Vocational Education and Technology*, *10*(2), 1–16. doi:10.4018/IJAVET.2019040101

Örnek, A., & Arslan, H. (2019). The Habit of Watching Television and Using Computer in Primary School Children. In G. Sarı (Ed.), *Handbook of Research on Children's Consumption of Digital Media* (pp. 209–222). IGI Global. doi:10.4018/978-1-5225-5733-3.ch015

Orr, L., Pigeon, K., Reyes, B., & Weekley, L. (2020). Defining and Promoting Student Well-Being. In S. Padmanaban & C. Subudhi (Eds.), *Psycho-Social Perspectives on Mental Health and Well-Being* (pp. 15–40). IGI Global. doi:10.4018/978-1-7998-1185-5.ch002

Orta, I. M., & Örücü, M. Ç. (2019). Psychological Benefits and Detrimental Effects of Online Social Networking. In R. T. Gopalan (Ed.), *Intimacy and Developing Personal Relationships in the Virtual World* (pp. 21–39). IGI Global. doi:10.4018/978-1-5225-4047-2.ch002

Pal, A., & Banerjee, S. (2019). Understanding Online Falsehood From the Perspective of Social Problem. In I. E. Chiluwa & S. A. Samoilenko (Eds.), *Handbook of Research on Deception, Fake News, and Misinformation Online* (pp. 1–17). IGI Global. doi:10.4018/978-1-5225-8535-0.ch001

Pal, K. (2019). Assessing the Impact of RFID Technology Solutions in Supply Chain Management. In D. Goyal, S. Balamurugan, S. Peng, & D. S. Jat (Eds.), *The IoT and the Next Revolutions Automating the World* (pp. 16–32). IGI Global. doi:10.4018/978-1-5225-9246-4.ch002

Palazzolo, A. N., & Pizzo, D. L. (2020). Elementary Service-Learning Project Example. In G. Salinitri (Ed.), *Handbook of Research on Leadership Experience for Academic Direction (LEAD) Programs for Student Success* (pp. 132–144). IGI Global. doi:10.4018/978-1-7998-2430-5.ch008

Palazzolo, A. N., & Pizzo, D. L. (2020). The Structure of the LEAD Program. In G. Salinitri (Ed.), *Handbook of Research on Leadership Experience for Academic Direction (LEAD) Programs for Student Success* (pp. 105–117). IGI Global. doi:10.4018/978-1-7998-2430-5.ch006

Pandey, S. (2018). An Empirical Study of the Indian IT Sector on Typologies of Workaholism as Predictors of HR Crisis. In V. Ahuja & S. Rathore (Eds.), *Multidisciplinary Perspectives on Human Capital and Information Technology Professionals* (pp. 202–224). IGI Global. doi:10.4018/978-1-5225-5297-0.ch011

Papadopoulos, H. (2018). Technological Advancements and Distortion of Notion of Place. In Optimizing Current Practices in E-Services and Mobile Applications (pp. 62-83). IGI Global. doi:10.4018/978-1-5225-5026-6.ch004

Papazissi, T., & Chatzinikolaou, F. (2021). Medical and Nursing Civil Liability and Ethics in the Provision of Health Services. In K. Dinas, S. Petousis, M. Kalder, & G. Mavromatidis (Eds.), *Handbook of Research on Oncological and Endoscopical Dilemmas in Modern Gynecological Clinical Practice* (pp. 365–374). IGI Global. doi:10.4018/978-1-7998-4213-2.ch025

Paul, M. A., & Teli, B. A. (2021). ADHD and Substance Abuse in Children and Adolescents. In R. T. Gopalan (Ed.), *New Developments in Diagnosing, Assessing, and Treating ADHD* (pp. 220–228). IGI Global. doi:10.4018/978-1-7998-5495-1.ch014

Pedigo, T. W., & Howell, G. L. (2019). Heart-Based Teaching. In K. Daniels & K. Billingsley (Eds.), *Creating Caring and Supportive Educational Environments for Meaningful Learning* (pp. 70–101). IGI Global. doi:10.4018/978-1-5225-5748-7.ch005

Perreault, M. F., & Perreault, G. P. (2020). Mobile Gaming Strategic Communication and Fear of Missing Out (FoMO) in Fan Culture. In R. A. Dunn (Ed.), *Multidisciplinary Perspectives on Media Fandom* (pp. 253–269). IGI Global. doi:10.4018/978-1-7998-3323-9.ch014

Petersen, N. J., & Pearson, R. L. (2020). Mobbability. In C. M. Crawford (Ed.), *Confronting Academic Mobbing in Higher Education* (pp. 104–131). IGI Global. doi:10.4018/978-1-5225-9485-7.ch005

Pizzuto, G. (2020). LEADing in a Different Way. In G. Salinitri (Ed.), *Handbook of Research on Leadership Experience for Academic Direction (LEAD) Programs for Student Success* (pp. 225–237). IGI Global. doi:10.4018/978-1-7998-2430-5.ch012

Plummer, B. A. (2019). Boring Into the State of Boredom Through Age Groups. In P. D. Keough (Ed.), *Ethical Problem-Solving and Decision-Making for Positive and Conclusive Outcomes* (pp. 57–77). IGI Global. doi:10.4018/978-1-5225-7582-5.ch004

Podgornik, N. (2019). A Psychosocial Approach to Treating Young People's and Young Adults' Computer Addictions. In B. Bozoglan (Ed.), *Multifaceted Approach to Digital Addiction and Its Treatment* (pp. 281–291). IGI Global. doi:10.4018/978-1-5225-8449-0.ch013

Prasath, P. R., & Copeland, L. (2021). Rationale and Benefits of Using Play Therapy and Expressive Art Techniques in Supervision. In L. J. Fazio-Griffith & R. Marino (Eds.), *Techniques and Interventions for Play Therapy and Clinical Supervision* (pp. 17–37). IGI Global. doi:10.4018/978-1-7998-4628-4.ch002

Priyadarshini, R., Malarvizhi, N., & Neeba, E. A. (2019). A Study on Capabilities and Challenges of Fog Computing. In P. Raj & S. Koteeswaran (Eds.), *Novel Practices and Trends in Grid and Cloud Computing* (pp. 249–273). IGI Global. doi:10.4018/978-1-5225-9023-1.ch015

Puaschunder, J. (2020). Towards a Utility Theory of Privacy and Information Sharing and the Introduction of Hyper-Hyperbolic Discounting in the Digital Big Data Age. In E. C. Idemudia (Ed.), *Handbook of Research on Social and Organizational Dynamics in the Digital Era* (pp. 157–200). IGI Global. doi:10.4018/978-1-5225-8933-4.ch008

Quinn, R. D., Arnold, A., & Littlewood, K. A. (2020). The Transformative Nature of Community Engagement in the Arts. In A. S. Zimmerman (Ed.), *Preparing Students for Community-Engaged Scholarship in Higher Education* (pp. 379–402). IGI Global. doi:10.4018/978-1-7998-2208-0.ch019

Radebe, J. (2021). The Ancient Wisdom and Resurgence for Yoga. In N. Mthembu (Ed.), *Ethical Research Approaches to Indigenous Knowledge Education* (pp. 206–227). IGI Global. doi:10.4018/978-1-7998-1249-4.ch009

Raman, K. (2021). Adolescents and Attention Deficit Hyperactivity Disorder (ADHD). In R. T. Gopalan (Ed.), *New Developments in Diagnosing, Assessing, and Treating ADHD* (pp. 70–87). IGI Global. doi:10.4018/978-1-7998-5495-1.ch005

Ramdeo, S., & Singh, R. (2020). Cyberbullying in the Workplace. In Encyclopedia of Criminal Activities and the Deep Web (pp. 686-698). IGI Global. doi:10.4018/978-1-5225-9715-5.ch047

Rao, D. S., & Kumar, A. (2020). Development and Validation of the Social Media Self-Esteem Scale for Adolescents. *International Journal of Cyber Behavior, Psychology and Learning*, *10*(4), 1–13. doi:10.4018/IJCBPL.2020100101

Rath, M. (2019). Resolution of Issues and Health Improvement Using Big Data and IoT. In G. Nagarajan & R. Minu (Eds.), *Edge Computing and Computational Intelligence Paradigms for the IoT* (pp. 216–237). IGI Global. doi:10.4018/978-1-5225-8555-8.ch013

Revell, M. D. (2021). Sustaining Culturally Responsive Teaching Practices. In K. Sprott, J. R. O'Connor Jr, & C. Msengi (Eds.), *Designing Culturally Competent Programming for PK-20 Classrooms* (pp. 218–239). IGI Global. doi:10.4018/978-1-7998-3652-0.ch012

Rivas, B. A., & Rivas, A. L. (2020). Causes and Implications of the Opioid Crisis in Rural America. In H. C. Greene, B. S. Zugelder, & J. C. Manner (Eds.), *Handbook of Research on Leadership and Advocacy for Children and Families in Rural Poverty* (pp. 46–74). IGI Global. doi:10.4018/978-1-7998-2787-0.ch003

Roysircar, G., Lanza, A. M., & Macedonia, M. F. (2020). Disaster Responder Self-Care, Self-Compassion, and Protective Factors. In Mental Health Intervention and Treatment of First Responders and Emergency Workers (pp. 169-189). IGI Global. http://doi:10.4018/978-1-5225-9803-9.ch010

Russell, L. D. (2020). Pervasive Technologies and Addiction. In S. Hai-Jew (Ed.), *Maintaining Social Well-Being and Meaningful Work in a Highly Automated Job Market* (pp. 125–144). IGI Global. doi:10.4018/978-1-7998-2509-8.ch005

Sabharwal, D. (2019). Study of Consumers' Attitudes Towards Marketing of Environmentally Friendly Products. In S. Narula, S. Rai, & A. Sharma (Eds.), *Environmental Awareness and the Role of Social Media* (pp. 150–168). IGI Global. doi:10.4018/978-1-5225-5291-8.ch008

Sağlam, H. (2019). Effects of Computer Games on the Socialization Process and Inclination to Violence of Adolescent Students. In G. Sarı (Ed.), *Handbook of Research on Children's Consumption of Digital Media* (pp. 235–257). IGI Global. doi:10.4018/978-1-5225-5733-3.ch017

Şahin, M. (2019). The Cognitive Emotional Behavioral and Physical Effects of Cartoons on Children. In G. Sarı (Ed.), *Handbook of Research on Children's Consumption of Digital Media* (pp. 323–342). IGI Global. doi:10.4018/978-1-5225-5733-3.ch022

Şahin, M., Keskin, S., & Yurdugül, H. (2019). Impact of Family Support and Perception of Loneliness on Game Addiction Analysis of a Mediation and Moderation. *International Journal of Game-Based Learning*, *9*(4), 15–30. doi:10.4018/IJGBL.2019100102

Samaha, M., & Hawi, N. (2020). Internet Gaming Disorder and Its Relationships With Student Engagement and Academic Performance. *International Journal of Cyber Behavior, Psychology and Learning*, *10*(4), 14–33. doi:10.4018/IJCBPL.2020100102

Samoilenko, S. A., & Miroshnichenko, A. (2019). Profiting From the "Trump Bump". In I. E. Chiluwa & S. A. Samoilenko (Eds.), *Handbook of Research on Deception, Fake News, and Misinformation Online* (pp. 375–391). IGI Global. doi:10.4018/978-1-5225-8535-0.ch020

Santaella, D. F. (2021). Neurobiology of Meditation. In S. Telles & R. K. Gupta (Eds.), *Handbook of Research on Evidence-Based Perspectives on the Psychophysiology of Yoga and Its Applications* (pp. 61–71). IGI Global. doi:10.4018/978-1-7998-3254-6.ch004

Saraç, M. (2020). A Literature Review on Mindfulness at Work Places. In E. Baykal (Ed.), *Handbook of Research on Positive Organizational Behavior for Improved Workplace Performance* (pp. 55–71). IGI Global. doi:10.4018/978-1-7998-0058-3.ch004

Sasso, M. T., & Ross, D. B. (2020). Academic Entitlement and the K-20 System. In J. R. O'Connor (Ed.), *Strategic Leadership in PK-12 Settings* (pp. 110–132). IGI Global. doi:10.4018/978-1-5225-9242-6.ch009

Sawyer-Kurian, K. M., & Coneal, W. B. (2018). The Double-Edged Sword of "Othermothering" for African American Women Faculty With Families. In C. S. Conway (Ed.), *Faculty Mentorship at Historically Black Colleges and Universities* (pp. 151–178). IGI Global. doi:10.4018/978-1-5225-4071-7.ch008

Scott, D. M. (2020). Hearing Loss and Diabetes in an African American Adult. In D. M. Scott (Ed.), *Cases on Communication Disorders in Culturally Diverse Populations* (pp. 280–297). IGI Global. doi:10.4018/978-1-7998-2261-5.ch014

Selzer, R. A., Srivastava, R., & Huckleberry, A. (2020). Using the Intercultural Development Inventory (IDI) With First-Year, Pre-Med Students. In R. Gotian, Y. Kang, & J. Safdieh (Eds.), *Handbook of Research on the Efficacy of Training Programs and Systems in Medical Education* (pp. 156–176). IGI Global. doi:10.4018/978-1-7998-1468-9.ch009

Sethi, K., Chauhan, S., & Jaiswal, V. (2021). Artificial Intelligence in Higher Education. In Impact of AI Technologies on Teaching, Learning, and Research in Higher Education (pp. 1-29). IGI Global. doi:10.4018/978-1-7998-4763-2.ch001

Sheely-Moore, A. I., & Daniel, A. (2021). Expressive Arts in Play Therapy Supervision for Substance Abuse Issues. In L. J. Fazio-Griffith & R. Marino (Eds.), *Techniques and Interventions for Play Therapy and Clinical Supervision* (pp. 38–55). IGI Global. doi:10.4018/978-1-7998-4628-4.ch003

Sheftel, I., & Sips, A. (2021). Neurocognitive Mechanisms of Yoga. In S. Telles & R. K. Gupta (Eds.), *Handbook of Research on Evidence-Based Perspectives on the Psychophysiology of Yoga and Its Applications* (pp. 124–142). IGI Global. doi:10.4018/978-1-7998-3254-6.ch008

Shen, L. (2019). Therapeutic Approaches for Internet Addiction. In B. Bozoglan (Ed.), *Multifaceted Approach to Digital Addiction and Its Treatment* (pp. 230–259). IGI Global. doi:10.4018/978-1-5225-8449-0.ch011

Shen, L., & Su, A. (2019). Intervention of Smartphone Addiction. In B. Bozoglan (Ed.), *Multifaceted Approach to Digital Addiction and Its Treatment* (pp. 207–228). IGI Global. doi:10.4018/978-1-5225-8449-0.ch010

Sice, P. V., Thirkle, S. A., & Ogwu, S. A. (2018). MIKE. *International Journal of Systems and Society*, *5*(1), 13–27. doi:10.4018/IJSS.2018010102

Sliwinski, J. (2019). Mindfulness and HCI. In K. Blashki & P. Isaías (Eds.), *Handbook of Research on Human-Computer Interfaces and New Modes of Interactivity* (pp. 314–332). IGI Global. doi:10.4018/978-1-5225-9069-9.ch018

Srivastava, A. P. (2018). Attrition Risk Management. In M. Yadav, S. Kumar Trivedi, A. Kumar, & S. Rangnekar (Eds.), *Harnessing Human Capital Analytics for Competitive Advantage* (pp. 91–112). IGI Global. doi:10.4018/978-1-5225-4038-0.ch004

Srivastava, G., & Tripathi, R. K. (2018). Sleep and Sleep Disorders in Old Age. In B. V. Prasad & S. Akbar (Eds.), *Handbook of Research on Geriatric Health, Treatment, and Care* (pp. 303–325). IGI Global. doi:10.4018/978-1-5225-3480-8.ch017

Stephen, D. J., & Rodriguez, M. (2020). Medical Education With Multicultural Perspectives. In L. O. Tripp & R. M. Collier (Eds.), *Culturally Responsive Teaching and Learning in Higher Education* (pp. 218–238). IGI Global. doi:10.4018/978-1-5225-9989-0.ch010

Stricker, A. G., & Calongne, C. (2019). Transformation and Development of Identity and Society With Virtual Learning. In A. G. Stricker, C. Calongne, B. Truman, & F. J. Arenas (Eds.), *Recent Advances in Applying Identity and Society Awareness to Virtual Learning* (pp. 1–26). IGI Global. doi:10.4018/978-1-5225-9679-0.ch001

Sumer, S. S. (2020). An Analysis of 100 Muslim Email Counseling Clients. In A. Bagasra & M. Mackinem (Eds.), *Working With Muslim Clients in the Helping Professions* (pp. 221–241). IGI Global. doi:10.4018/978-1-7998-0018-7.ch012

Tarai, S. (2019). Neurocognitive Mechanisms for Detecting Early Phase of Depressive Disorder. In S. Paul, P. Bhattacharya, & A. Bit (Eds.), *Early Detection of Neurological Disorders Using Machine Learning Systems* (pp. 165–198). IGI Global. doi:10.4018/978-1-5225-8567-1.ch010

Tebay, G. (2019). Cultivating Compassion in an Upper Elementary School Classroom Community. In V. Bohac Clarke (Ed.), *Integral Theory and Transdisciplinary Action Research in Education* (pp. 160–181). IGI Global. doi:10.4018/978-1-5225-5873-6.ch008

Terras, M. M., & Ramsay, J. (2019). Mobile Use During Adolescence. In X. Xu (Ed.), *Impacts of Mobile Use and Experience on Contemporary Society* (pp. 1–19). IGI Global. doi:10.4018/978-1-5225-7885-7.ch001

Thirkle, S. A., Kennedy, A., & Sice, P. (2018). A Case for TIC. *International Journal of Systems and Society, 5*(2), 1–12. doi:10.4018/IJSS.2018070101

Tomar, R. S., & Kulkarni, M. (2020). Global Racial, Ethnic, and Religious Subculture and Its Impact on Healthcare Organizations. In M. Merviö (Ed.), *Global Issues and Innovative Solutions in Healthcare, Culture, and the Environment* (pp. 253–270). IGI Global. doi:10.4018/978-1-7998-3576-9.ch013

Travis, F. (2021). Negative and Positive Mind-Wandering. In M. R. Gurubatham & G. A. Williams (Eds.), *Advancing Innovation and Sustainable Outcomes in International Graduate Education* (pp. 177–192). IGI Global. doi:10.4018/978-1-7998-5514-9.ch011

Ulusoy, Ş. G. (2019). Communication Disorders That Tablet Usage Causes in Children in the Age Group 9 to 12 Years. In G. Sarı (Ed.), *Handbook of Research on Children's Consumption of Digital Media* (pp. 156–176). IGI Global. doi:10.4018/978-1-5225-5733-3.ch012

Ünal, A. T. (2021). Aesthetics Perceptions of Social Media Generations. In M. N. Erdem, N. Kocabay-Sener, & T. Demir (Eds.), *Handbook of Research on Aestheticization of Violence, Horror, and Power* (pp. 543–566). IGI Global. doi:10.4018/978-1-7998-4655-0.ch027

Ursu, A. S., Panisoara, I. O., & Chirca, R. C. (2021). The Changes Brought by Digital Technology to Cognitive Learning. In J. Pelet (Ed.), *Handbook of Research on User Experience in Web 2.0 Technologies and Its Impact on Universities and Businesses* (pp. 161–182). IGI Global. doi:10.4018/978-1-7998-3756-5.ch010

Uzbay, T. (2020). Importance of Brain Reward System in Neuromarketing. In D. Atli (Ed.), *Analyzing the Strategic Role of Neuromarketing and Consumer Neuroscience* (pp. 1–24). IGI Global. doi:10.4018/978-1-7998-3126-6.ch001

Vidourek, R. A., & King, K. A. (2019). Preventing Teen Pregnancy Among Minority Populations. In D. Akella (Ed.), *Socio-Cultural Influences on Teenage Pregnancy and Contemporary Prevention Measures* (pp. 189–207). IGI Global. doi:10.4018/978-1-5225-6108-8.ch011

Villetto, D. A. (2019). It's Nice to Be Nice. In N. R. Silton (Ed.), *Scientific Concepts Behind Happiness, Kindness, and Empathy in Contemporary Society* (pp. 76–89). IGI Global. doi:10.4018/978-1-5225-5918-4.ch004

Webster, T. E. (2018). On Being Earnest. *International Journal of Computer-Assisted Language Learning and Teaching, 8*(4), 1–12. doi:10.4018/IJCALLT.2018100101

Webster, T. E. (2020). The Need to Engage With Smartphones and Social Network Sites (SNSs) at Korean Universities. In B. Zou & M. Thomas (Eds.), *Recent Developments in Technology-Enhanced and Computer-Assisted Language Learning* (pp. 122–143). IGI Global. doi:10.4018/978-1-7998-1282-1.ch006

Wickramasinghe, N. (2020). Minority Health and Wellness. In N. Wickramasinghe (Ed.), *Handbook of Research on Optimizing Healthcare Management Techniques* (pp. 116–126). IGI Global. doi:10.4018/978-1-7998-1371-2.ch008

Wienhold-Leahy, B. (2019). An Integral Analysis of Mindfulness and Self-Compassion Among Adolescents. In V. Bohac Clarke (Ed.), *Integral Theory and Transdisciplinary Action Research in Education* (pp. 134–159). IGI Global. doi:10.4018/978-1-5225-5873-6.ch007

Williams, Y. (2021). An Exploration of ADHD and Comorbidity With Substance Abuse and Brain Development. In R. T. Gopalan (Ed.), *New Developments in Diagnosing, Assessing, and Treating ADHD* (pp. 245–258). IGI Global. doi:10.4018/978-1-7998-5495-1.ch016

Wong, P. T., & Bowers, V. (2019). Mature Happiness and Global Wellbeing in Difficult Times. In N. R. Silton (Ed.), *Scientific Concepts Behind Happiness, Kindness, and Empathy in Contemporary Society* (pp. 112–134). IGI Global. doi:10.4018/978-1-5225-5918-4.ch006

Wright, K. (2018). Show Me What You Are Saying. In A. August (Ed.), *Visual Imagery, Metadata, and Multimodal Literacies Across the Curriculum* (pp. 24–49). IGI Global. doi:10.4018/978-1-5225-2808-1.ch002

Xu, H. D. (2020). Health Challenges for Rural Families. In H. C. Greene, B. S. Zugelder, & J. C. Manner (Eds.), *Handbook of Research on Leadership and Advocacy for Children and Families in Rural Poverty* (pp. 1–22). IGI Global. doi:10.4018/978-1-7998-2787-0.ch001

Ye, P., Liu, L., Gao, L., & Mei, Q. (2020). Factors Affecting Woman's Continuance Intention for Mobile Games. *International Journal of Information and Communication Technology Education, 16*(4), 48–67. doi:10.4018/IJICTE.2020100104

Yeşiltaş, M., & Gürlek, M. (2020). Understanding the Nature of Deviant Workplace Behaviors. In Ş. Aydin, B. B. Dedeoglu, & Ö. Çoban (Eds.), *Organizational Behavior Challenges in the Tourism Industry* (pp. 305–326). IGI Global. doi:10.4018/978-1-7998-1474-0.ch017

Yildirim, S. (2020). Examining Perceived Value Influence Mobile Game Addiction. In Leveraging Consumer Behavior and Psychology in the Digital Economy (pp. 133-152). IGI Global. http://doi:10.4018/978-1-7998-3042-9.ch008

Zaleski, J. R., & Peruvemba, R. (2019). The Analytic Link Between Population Health and Leading Hospital and Ambulatory Patient Safety Considerations. In G. W. Evans, W. E. Biles, & K. G. Bae (Eds.), *Analytics, Operations, and Strategic Decision Making in the Public Sector* (pp. 111–136). IGI Global. doi:10.4018/978-1-5225-7591-7.ch006

Zarcadoolas, C., & Kondilis, B. K. (2018). Health Literacy in Non-Communicable Diseases. In V. E. Papalois & M. Theodosopoulou (Eds.), *Optimizing Health Literacy for Improved Clinical Practices* (pp. 32–72). IGI Global. doi:10.4018/978-1-5225-4074-8.ch003

Zbinden, B. (2019). Restricted Communication. In L. Oliveira & D. Graça (Eds.), *Infocommunication Skills as a Rehabilitation and Social Reintegration Tool for Inmates* (pp. 238–267). IGI Global. doi:10.4018/978-1-5225-5975-7.ch011

Zhao, Y., & Wang, Y. (2018). Mediated Hook-Up. *International Journal of Cyber Behavior, Psychology and Learning, 8*(3), 48–64. doi:10.4018/IJCBPL.2018070105

Ziemendorf, A. L., & Schroyer, S. (2020). Supporting the Spiritual Experience in Online Faith-Based Education. In L. Kyei-Blankson, E. Ntuli, & J. Blankson (Eds.), *Handbook of Research on Creating Meaningful Experiences in Online Courses* (pp. 270–285). IGI Global. doi:10.4018/978-1-7998-0115-3.ch016

About the Author

Cheryl Green, PhD, DNP, RN, LCSW, CNL, CNE, ACUE, MAC, FAPA, has been a registered nurse for over 31 years and a licensed clinical social worker for over 27 years. Her areas of research include: mental illness, medication error prevention, simulation, incivility and discrimination, prayer and spirituality, self-care, stress, distraction and anxiety, health disparities, medical and surgical health issues, diversity and equity within nursing education, complementary alternative approaches to stress reduction in nursing students, and mindfulness. She has served as a board member and committee chair of university and professional organizations, most recently the Connecticut Nurses Association, the Connecticut League of Nursing, and the Connecticut National Association of Social Workers. Dr. Green provides dissertation/thesis supervision at the master's and doctoral levels and teaches undergraduate and graduate nursing students. She is also an Off-Shift Nurse Leader at Yale-New Haven Hospital and Associate Professor of Nursing at Southern Connecticut State University.

Index

Printed in the United States
by Baker & Taylor Publisher Services